CW00921139

OXFORD MEDICAL PUBL

The Art of General Practice

The Art of General Practice

DAVID MORRELL

Wolfson Professor of General Practice,
United Medical and Dental Schools of Guy's and
St Thomas's Hospitals, London

Oxford   New York   Tokyo
OXFORD UNIVERSITY PRESS
1991

Oxford University Press, Walton Street, Oxford OX2 6DP
Oxford   New York   Toronto
Delhi   Bombay   Calcutta   Madras   Karachi
Petaling Jaya   Singapore   Hong Kong   Tokyo
Nairobi   Dar es Salaam   Cape Town
Melbourne   Auckland

and associated companies in
Berlin   Ibadan

Oxford is a trade mark of Oxford University Press

Published in the United States
by Oxford University Press, New York

First edition published 1965 with the title The Art of General Practice by
E. and S. Livingstone
Second edition published 1976 with the title An Introduction to Primary
Medical Care by E. and S. Livingstone
Third edition published 1981 with the title An Introduction to Primary
Medical Care (2nd edn) by Churchill Livingstone
This edition published 1991 by Oxford University Press

© David Morrell, 1991

British Library Cataloguing in Publication Data
Morrell, D. C. (David Cameron)
The Art of general practice.—4th. ed.
1. Great Britain. General practice
I. Title
362.1720941
ISBN 0–19–261988–8
ISBN 0–19–261990–X (pbk)

Library of Congress Cataloging in Publication Data
Morrell, David Cameron.
[4th ed.]
The art of general practice / David Morrell.
p.   cm.
Rev. ed. of: An introduction to primary medical care. 3rd ed.
1981.
Includes index.
1. Family medicine. I. Title.
[DNLM: 1. Family Practice. 2. Primary Health Care. W 89 M873a]
RC48.M597 1991   616—dc20   90–7962
ISBN 0–19–261988–8
ISBN 0–19–261990–X (pbk)

Set by Footnote Graphics, Warminster, Wiltshire
Printed in Great Britain by Bookcraft, Midsomer Norton, Avon

Preface

In 1965 E. and S. Livingstone published my first book entitled *The Art of General Practice*. I wrote this during my first five years in general practice in an attempt to describe how I struggled to adapt the knowledge that I had acquired in training to the problems encountered in general practice. It was designed to help new doctors entering general practice. The book was warmly received by the profession and to extend its international appeal, it was renamed *An Introduction to Primary Medical Care* in the second and third editions. Although originally planned to satisfy the needs of new entrants to general practice, it became increasingly popular among medical students and has been used as a course book throughout the world.

The decision to republish the book ten years after the last edition is based primarily on a still-evident need for a text of this type for undergraduates undertaking studies in general practice. It is designed to help them relate their experience of hospital medicine to the practice of primary medical care. Many of these problems will also be experienced by trainee general practitioners. The book is written in the context of the British National Health Service, but the knowledge and skills demanded of general practitioners throughout the world have much in common, despite the detailed differences in the organization of care. It is hoped that this new edition will attract the international enthusiasm of previous editions.

Several textbooks on general practice have been written for medical students, but none of these combine the scientific approach based on the author's own research with the case histories that have characterized this book and proved so popular in the past. This book adheres to this format but contains a large amount of new material.

The first chapter tackles the problems of teaching and learning in general practice, spelling out the aims of undergraduate teaching in general practice and relating this to opportunities for learning in hospital. There are two new chapters describing the organization and characteristics of primary care. The book then reverts to the original pattern, describing with numerous examples, the special skills needed for problem solving, history taking, physical examination, and making a prognosis in general practice. New chapters are introduced on prevention and the primary care team, and the chapter on treatment has been extended to consider continuing care for chronic diseases and terminal care.

To mark a major change in emphasis in this book, it was decided to revert to the original title, *The Art of General Practice*. This change reflects, perhaps, a change in the perspective of the author. Twenty-five years ago, I was keen to establish the scientific respectability of general practice. Today, though no less convinced that scientific rigour is as important in primary as in secondary care, I have come to realize that it is something more than this, something much less easily measured, which characterizes the effective general practitioner.

Art is defined in the *Shorter Oxford Dictionary* as 'skill as the result of knowledge and practice'. In reflecting on the accepted arts such as painting or music, it is clear that the artist is using knowledge, be this of colour, melody, timing, or perspective and expressing these by constant practice through physical skills to create an impression and achieve an objective. Art is usually concerned with creating an ambience, delivering a message, and expecting an emotional response.

What then is the art of general practice? Effective general practitioners develop their knowledge and skills from a wide variety of basic and clinical sciences. They should retain, throughout their professional lives, a scientific approach to new knowledge including that which they derive from their own personal experience. Their skills include the ability to listen, to observe, to examine, and to interpret what they hear and see; to communicate and share with their patients their thoughts, conclusions, and advice; to establish a relationship that, at different times, is diagnostic, therapeutic, or supportive. In this they must create an ambience and involve their 'audience', the patients.

Some of their skills may be taught and learned. Others come from constant practice, wherein they become able to adapt them to different clinical situations, to the needs of different individuals with different personalities and social backgrounds. The outcome of their work may be measured in terms of cure, care, compliance, or patient satisfaction, but the process that achieves desirable outcomes is dependent on more than the application of knowledge in physical, psychological, and social terms.

Does this differ from medical practice in the hospital setting? The answer to this is usually 'Yes'. The reason for this difference is that the ease of access that patients have to the general practitioner leads to the production of an infinitely wide variety of problems and the continuing relationship between general practitioner and patient that often spans many years.

To describe the 'art' of general practice as 'skill as the result of knowledge and practice' reflects, for many doctors, the greatest source of satisfaction in their work. In the pursuit of scientific knowledge, the art has sometimes been ignored. This book attempts to redress the balance.

London
October 1990   D.M.

Contents

1

Teaching and learning in general practice

It is a sound educational principle that in undertaking any educational project, teachers should clearly define what they expect the student to learn as a result of their efforts. The General Medical Council in the United Kingdom has clearly stated the objectives of medical education (GMC 1980). It has been argued that many of these cannot be achieved effectively without medical students spending some time in general practice (Royal College of General Practitioners 1984). Examples of some GMC objectives that are relevant to medical education throughout the world include:

1. To acquire knowledge and understanding of:
    (c) The aetiology, natural history and prognosis of the common mental and physical ailments. Students must have experience of emergencies, and good knowledge of the commoner disabling diseases and of ageing processes.
    (e) The principles of prevention and of therapy including health education, the amelioration of suffering and disability, rehabilitation, the maintenance of health in old age, and the care of the dying.
    (f) Human relationships, both personal and communal, and the interaction between man and his physical, biological and social environment.
    (g) The organisation and provision of health care in the community and in hospital; the identification of the need for it, and the economic, ethical and practical constraints within which it operates.
    (h) The ethical standards and legal responsibilities of the medical profession.
2. To develop the professional skills necessary:
    (a) To elicit, record and interpret the relevant medical history, symptoms and physical signs, and to identify the problems and how these may be managed.
    (e) To communicate clinical information accurately and concisely, both by word of mouth and in writing to medical colleagues and to other professionals involved in the care of the patient.

3. To develop appropriate attitudes to the practice of medicine, which include:
   (a) Recognition that a blend of scientific and humanitarian approaches is needed in medicine.
   (c) The ability to assess the reliability of evidence and the relevance of scientific knowledge, to reach conclusions by logical deduction or by experiment, and to evaluate critically methods and standards of medical practice.
   (f) The achievement of good working relationships with members of the other health care professions.

LEARNING IN GENERAL PRACTICE

Medical education is concerned with the acquisition of a large amount of scientific knowledge and skills; the ability to acquire such knowledge being closely related to motivation. Students may derive their motivation from accepting that such knowledge is essential if they are to undertake certain tasks or fulfil a certain career. But a much more potent source of motivation for them is to recognize that such knowledge is important if they are to cope with the everyday challenges that form part of the educational system. In the case of medicine, these challenges are concerned with the day-to-day contact with patients. This contact also involves developing personal relationships with patients and recognizing and handling their emotional concerns, which provides a further stimulus to learning. Furthermore, the apprenticeship system of learning that is widely used in general practice, provokes the student into attempting to solve problems that are presented by patients, thus transforming the pure acquisition of knowledge and skills into an intellectual activity in which the knowledge acquired is used to interpret and, it is hoped, solve clinical problems. General practice provides an environment in which the medical student can come face to face with the problems of providing primary medical care. In this situation, the student will inevitably be faced with: defining normality when dealing with the early stages of illness; understanding the factors that influence individuals in deciding to seek medical care; appreciating the patterns of morbidity in the community and the probability of disease in the presence of symptoms of illness; the difference between illness, disease, and disability; the importance of communication between patients and doctors in identifying problems and in the management of illness; the importance of a primary care team of professionals in providing continuing care; and the importance of health education and prevention.

All these issues are important to the student who wishes to have a proper understanding of medicine and its role in the community. The knowledge acquired in general practice complements that learned in hospitals, but it also introduces new concepts of disease and disability, because for the first time the student observes illness occurring in its natural environment and can appreciate the potential for health education and prevention in the community setting. It also becomes apparent that the information required to solve clinical problems, the methods of problem-solving employed, and the way illness is managed, are different in general practice.

This book is designed to help students integrate what they observe and experience in general practice into their medical education. In learning in general practice, the patients are the most effective teachers. The main role of tutors of general practice is to act as catalysts encouraging and facilitating interchange between student and patient. The written word helps to interpret these exchanges and to make explicit that which remains unsaid and unappreciated in general practice, which can sometimes be an intense and pressurized environment.

Experience in general practice and primary medical care varies between medical schools. Many students get an early opportunity to meet patients in the community during their first or second year by attachment to general practitioners for half or single days. This is primarily intended to provide experience some of the problems encountered in medical care and to give relevance to courses in anatomy, physiology, pharmacology, sociology, and psychology. In some medical schools, departments of general practice play a major part in teaching communication skills. Indeed, they are often instrumental in introducing such courses to the curriculum. In nearly all schools, a more substantial time of 1–2 months is spent in general practice when the student, attached to a selected practice, acquires clinical experience in the delivery of medical care. Such courses are often backed up by seminar teaching to provide an opportunity for the feedback of practical experience to a group and, through discussion, to determine the general principles governing the provision of medical care.

In some schools, students are invited either individually or in groups to develop projects in which they study certain aspects of medical care in more depth. This demands intellectual initiatives, literature reviews, and, in some cases, the collection and interpretation of data. This brings home the fact that the knowledge on which medical practice depends is constantly changing and that a critical approach is essential in those who will practise medicine into the next century.

REFERENCES

General Medical Council (1980). *Recommendations on basic medical education*. GMC, London.

Royal College of General Practitioners (1984). Undergraduate medical education in general practice. *Journal of the Royal College of General Practitioners*, Occasional Paper 28.

2

Primary medical care

Although it is unnecessary for the undergraduate to have detailed knowledge of the organization of primary care services, it is useful to have some understanding of the framework within which these services work. More importantly, the basic philosophy that under-lies the development of primary care determines many of the characteristics of general practice and the problems that are pre-sented to and managed by general practitioners. This philosophy has led to certain principles that have determined the way in which services have developed. The principles developed in the United Kingdom are summarized below and the influence that they have had on the content and the clinical method in general practice will be considered later.

General practitioner care in the United Kingdom is designed to ensure that:

1. Every individual in the community has the right to register with a general practitioner for primary medical care services.

2. This doctor provides the normal point of entry to medical care in the National Health Service (exceptions occur in the case of accidents and emergencies).

3. While individuals are free to change their general practitioner, they cannot be registered with more than one general practi-tioner at any point in time.

4. The general practitioner has responsibility for maintaining a record of the care provided and for transferring this record to the next general practitioner if the individual changes doctor.

5. Individuals are encouraged to remain registered with the same doctor over a period of time to ensure continuity of care.

6. The general practitioner maintains his statutory responsibility for providing all necessary care and in so doing refers individuals to

secondary facilities—that is, hospital care, which in the National Health Service is normally arranged through the general practitioner—when necessary.

7. Responsibility for the care of an individual admitted to hospital is transferred back to the general practitioner on discharge, even if the individual continues to attend the out-patient department of the hospital. The term consultant, when applied to specialists, means what it implies—that is, one who is consulted by the general practitioner and the patient.

8. All medical care in the National Health Service is provided free at the time of delivery and is paid for mainly from general taxation.

9. Individuals are free to seek private general practitioner care. This contributes less than 5 per cent of primary care services, however, which might reflect general satisfaction with the services already provided. Secondary care may also be obtained privately, but most specialists respect the role of the general practitioner and will only see individuals privately in response to a letter of referral.

INTERNATIONAL VARIATIONS

The essential principles of general practice are the same throughout the world, being concerned with the provision of personal, primary, and continuing care. Methods of financing primary care, however, differ in different countries. Primary care in the United Kingdom is similar to that in Scandinavia, the Netherlands, Canada, Australia, and New Zealand, but the financing is variously provided by health insurance, government finance derived from taxation, or a mixture of both. Methods of payment vary between a capitation system and payment for the services rendered. The contribution of general practitioners to hospital care also varies, for example, in Canada and the United States many general practitioners enjoy what are described as 'hospital privileges', that is, they provide care for their patients in hospital, whereas in the United Kingdom this only occurs in small community hospitals. Though the differences in the financing of primary care inevitably influence the way in which care is delivered and the nature of the doctor-patient relationship, they have little influence on the knowledge and skills that are demanded of general practitioners throughout the world and described in this book.

OTHER SOURCES OF PRIMARY CARE

Primary care services are not limited to medical care, but include dental, ophthalmic, and pharmaceutical services. In addition, the provision of primary care in the community also involves the provision of nursing, health visiting, midwifery, and a variety of social services.

ORGANIZATION OF PRIMARY CARE

Three administrative bodies are responsible for delivering primary care in the United Kingdom. Firstly, there are the family health services authorities. There are 98 such authorities throughout the country and they are responsible for ensuring that there are general practitioner, ophthalmic, dental, and pharmaceutical services available in their area of jurisdiction. These authorities are composed of professional and lay members who determine an overall policy that is then carried out by a chief executive, supported by appropriate staff. All professionals providing primary care services are independent contractors of a family health service authority, which means that they are paid through an authority on the basis of the population they serve. For general practitioners this depends on the number of patients registered with the practice and on payments for some of the services delivered. Pharmacists, ophthalmic practitioners, and dentists are paid entirely on the basis of the items of service they provide.

It might be expected that these authorities would experience difficulties in ensuring an equitable distribution of general practitioners throughout the country. This is not so, however, because regulations exist that control the number of general practitioners who can work in any given area. Authorities have discretion in accepting general practitioners into an area that is over-doctored and inducement allowances can be paid to attract doctors to under-doctored areas. The overall distribution of doctors throughout

the United Kingdom is controlled by the Medical Practices
Committee of the British Medical Association, to which the
authorities must apply if they wish to vary the ratio of doctors to
potential patients in a given area. Similar checks and balances
control the distribution of pharmacists, ophthalmic practitioners,
and dentists.

Secondly, there are health authorities, of which there are 200 in
the country and their major concern is to ensure the provision of
secondary care services. They also control the distribution of community nurses, health visitors, and midwives who ideally should
work in association with general practitioners. In many health
authorities this occurs, but in others these professionals are responsible for geographical areas that are unrelated to the patients
registered with the general practitioners. Professional relationships based on a common concern for a defined community of
patients related to general practice are therefore more difficult to
develop. Health authorities are also responsible for the development of community care resources for patients discharged from
chronic mental institutions into the community. The needs of these
patients are closely related to social support and continuing primary

Table 2.1. Division of responsibility for care for the three
administrative bodies responsible for delivering primary care in
the United Kingdom

Family health services authority	District health authority	Local government
General practitioners	Hospital services	Housing
Ophthalmic practitioners	Public health medicine	Social services
Dental practitioners	District nurses	Environmental health
Pharmacists	District health visitors	Meals on wheels
	District midwives	Home help
	Residential care for mentally ill	Day care for elderly
	Chiropody	
	Community physiotherapy	
	Community psychiatric nurses	

care, and this situation is increasingly becoming the responsibility of local authorities.

Local authorities are the third administrative body responsible for delivering primary care in the United Kingdom. They are responsible for the provision of housing, social services, and environmental health. They provide facilities such as day care for the elderly, meals-on-wheels, home help services, social workers, and accommodation for the elderly and disabled. The division of responsibility for the care of the elderly, the chronic mentally sick, and those problems arising from environmental disadvantage, is thus shared between the health authorities, the local authorities, and the family health services authorities. These divisions are summarized in Table 2.1.

HOW TO BE A PATIENT IN THE NATIONAL HEALTH SERVICE

The day-to-day work of the National Health Service in providing care for individuals and families is summarized by the experiences of a typical family.

Mr and Mrs North recently married. They moved into a flat on the Nonesuch Estate. When Mrs North became pregnant, she decided that it was time that they registered with a general practitioner and she took their medical cards to Dr West, who had been recommended by a neighbour. His consulting rooms were over a mile away, but on her first visit to Dr West, when he confirmed her pregnancy, she thought that this had been a good choice. Dr West ran an appointment system and so she only had to wait a short while before being seen. He explained that he ran a special antenatal clinic and would provide all her antenatal care and arrange for her delivery in the local general practitioner obstetric unit. At her second antenatal visit, she met the specialist obstetrician who had overall responsiblity for obstetrics in the area. She was happy that she would be delivered either by her own general practitioner or by one of midwives working in his practice. She enjoyed her pregnancy, during which she got to know the practice health visitor, and she had an uncomplicated delivery. When the health visitor visited her 2 weeks after delivery, the health visitor suggested that she should attend the practice well-baby clinic with her new baby. This presented problems because there was no public transport from her home to the practice. She was told by her neighbours that Dr South provided a well-baby clinic in the next road to her house and so, with some regret, she decided to change her doctor. To do this she took her medical card to Dr South who accepted her and the baby on to his list.

When her baby was 6 weeks old, she visited Dr South for a postnatal examination and for the first examination of her baby. This was arranged by the health visitor attached to Dr South's practice. At the end of the consultation Dr South provided her with contraceptive advice and agreed to supervise her contraceptive care over the next year, for which he would receive a special payment. The geographical proximity of Dr South's practice made it easy for her to attend regularly for supervision of her baby's development and immunizations, and through these regular contacts with the doctor, the health visitor, and the nurse, Mrs North felt that she belonged to the practice and would have no difficulty in talking to the staff about her medical problems.

Three months later, her brother came to stay. He suffered from asthma and developed a severe attack during the night. She called Dr South who provided treatment, but asked her to sign a form stating that treatment had been delivered to a person temporarily resident in the neighbourhood. He explained that he would be paid for this service and that the record of treatment would be forwarded to her brother's normal practitioner. As he was called out at night, Dr South explained that he would also receive a special fee for a night visit.

Six months later, Mrs North's mother, Mrs East, who lived locally and was registered with Dr South's practice, had a stroke. Dr South cared for her at home, with the community nurses visiting daily and happily she made a good recovery, but had marked weakness in her right arm and leg and could only just cope with independent life in her flat. Dr South arranged for the local authority to provide a home help service and a bath attendant. To avoid her becoming socially isolated, he arranged for her to be taken by ambulance to a local lunch-club run by the local authority twice weekly. As a result of her stroke, she had problems with cutting her toenails and Dr South arranged regular visits to the local health authority chiropody service.

Although Mr and Mrs North and Mrs East did not have any appreciable financial resources, they felt that the National Health Service was providing comprehensive health care for their needs. Later, however, when Mr North required surgical treatment for a hernia and Mrs East needed a vaginal repair to correct her uterine prolapse and stress incontinence, they found that they had to wait over a year for treatment. Furthermore, when Mr North's mother became senile some months later and started walking the streets at night in her underwear, the shortcomings of the services provided became even more apparent.

In the provision of day-to-day primary care, they agreed that the National Health Service was capable of delivering one of the best services in the world, but that this care depended on the commitment and vocational ideals of individual general practitioners. In the provision of non-acute surgical treatment, however, it was far less satisfactory.

Care of the rapidly expanding elderly population is presenting problems throughout the western world and, though the National Health Service does better than many of the services in other countries, it still falls far short of meeting the needs of the population. This case history also illustrates the wide variety of demands that may be made on the National Health Service, which is committed to providing comprehensive care. It illustrates general practitioners' statutory responsibility in responding to requests for health care from all those individuals registered with them, and shows that they are expected to provide continuity of care for those suffering from chronic disease and to refer patients to the secondary care services when necessary. The effect of providing such an accessible service and continuity of care, and the knowledge and skills that doctors must possess to undertake their tasks, are described in the next chapters.

3

The characteristics of general practice

ACCESSIBILITY

One of the principles on which the health service in the United Kingdom has been built is that every individual may register with a general practitioner who should be accessible 24 hours a day and 365 days a year. If the general practitioner is not personally accessible, he or she must make the necessary arrangements to ensure that a deputy can be contacted. The decision to seek care from a general practitioner is a lay one, and depends on individuals deciding that they need the services of a doctor. The factors that influence this decision are crucial both to the workload of general practitioners and to the content of their work, and they have been the subject of some research.

Random samples of patients have been asked to recall the presence or absence of particular symptoms over defined periods of time, such as 2 weeks (Dunnell and Cartwright 1972) (see Table 3.1). This study showed that adults experienced symptoms of illness about every 4 days, but only a small proportion of these symptoms led to a consultation with a doctor. One of my studies, in which patients recorded their perceived symptoms of illness in health diaries, showed that symptoms were recorded on about one day in three (Morrell and Wale 1976). Fifty-seven per cent of these symptoms led to some form of self-medication and 18 per cent to some restriction of daily activities, but only 1 in 37 symptoms led to a consultation with the doctor. The action taken in response to common symptoms of illness is shown in Table 3.2.

A comparison of the relative frequency of symptoms recorded in health diaries and symptoms presented to the doctor for a sample of women patients in general practice is illustrated in Tables 3.3 and 3.4. From these tables it is clear that the probability of a symptom, perceived and recorded by a patient, leading to a

Table 3.1.   Symptoms reported by adults and children in a 2 week
period. From Dunnell and Cartwright (1972)

Symptom presented	Percentage reporting symptoms in a 2 week period	
	Adults	Children
Sore Throat	12	8
Breathlessness	15	1
Coughs, catarrh, or phlegm	32	17
Cold, 'flu, or running nose	18	18
Constipation	10	6
Diarrhoea	3	3
Vomiting	3	6
Indigestion	18	1
Eye strain or other eye trouble	14	4
Ear trouble	7	3
Faintness or dizziness	8	1
Headaches	38	8
Pain or trouble on passing water	2	–
Loss of appetite	6	4
Any problem of being underweight or overweight	10	–
'Nerves', depression, or irritability	21	3
Pains in the chest	5	–
Backache or pains in the back	21	1
Aches or pains in the joints, muscles, legs, or arms	29	3
Palpitations or thumping heart	6	–
Piles	5	–
Sores or ulcers	4	2
Rashes, itches, or other skin troubles	13	12
Sleeplessness	8	1
Burns, bruises, cuts, or other accidents	9	16
Trouble with teeth or gums	7	12
Undue tiredness	16	2
Corns, bunions, or any trouble with feet	19	2
Women's complaints (recorded only for females aged ≥10 years)	5	1
'A temperature'	2	3
Any other symptoms	6	3
Total number of people	1410	519
Average number of symptoms reported	3.9	1.4

Table 3.2. Action taken in response to the 12 most common symptoms reported in health diaries. From Morrell and Wale (1976)

Symptom	Total no. of days on which symptoms recorded	No. (%) days on which normal activities restricted	No. (%) days on which patient had to lie down	No. (%) days on which some form medication taken
Headache	365	54 (15)	58 (16)	252 (69)
Changes in energy or tiredness	207	54 (26)	60 (29)	84 (41)
Backache	143	24 (17)	33 (23)	54 (38)
Cold	128	31 (24)	20 (16)	80 (62)
Disturbance of gastric function	100	7 (7)	16 (16)	42 (42)
Disturbance of emotional response	100	21 (21)	12 (12)	61 (61)
Sore throat	90	17 (19)	14 (16)	53 (59)
Abdominal pain	88	19 (22)	18 (20)	46 (52)
Cough	74	20 (27)	14 (19)	60 (81)
Pain in the mouth (toothache)	55	4 (7)	1 (2)	45 (82)
Bleeding and abnormal discharge from nose	50	8 (16)	3 (6)	32 (64)
Disturbance of menstruation	48	11 (23)	11 (23)	28 (58)
Total symptom days	2027	366 (18)	333 (16)	1157 (57)

Table 3.3.   Symptom episodes from the diaries of 204 patients. From Morrell and Wale (1976)

Symptom episode recorded	number
Headache	294
Changes in energy	146
Backache	85
Disturbance of gastric function	71
Disturbance of emotional response	69
Abdominal pain	63
Sore throat	46
Cold	40
Pain in lower limb	36
Disturbance of menstruation	32
Others	385
Total	1267

consultation varies with the particular symptom recorded. This is predictable because some symptoms provoke more anxiety than others. Extensive research has shown that factors other than the symptom presented also influence the likelihood of a patient consulting a doctor. Objective measures of anxiety and depression have been shown to influence the propensity, not only to record symptoms but also to consult the doctor. Those individuals who score high on questionnaires designed to measure anxiety and depression are more likely both to record and report symptoms.

Education plays a part in determining behaviour in response to symptoms. Those who have received a higher education are less likely to consult a doctor in response to new symptoms than those of low educational attainment, but they are more likely to use preventive services. Women who have poor living conditions, who have lived a comparatively short time in a community, and who are dissatisfied with the community in which they live, are more likely to consult than those who are more established in the community and more satisfied with their housing. Available family support influences the propensity to consult. Mothers of large families are less likely to accept the sick role and consult the doctor

Table 3.4. Symptoms presented at 436 consultations in one year
initiated by 204 patients keeping health diaries.
From Morrell and Wale (1976)

Symptoms presented	Number
Sore throat	33
Cough	29
Abdominal pain	28
Skin rash	22
Disturbance of menstruation	21
Backache	21
Headache	20
Disturbance of bladder function	19
Bleeding or abnormal discharge from genital tract	16
Disturbance of bowel function	14
Chest pain	14
Disturbance of emotional response	14
Others	185
Total	436

than are mothers of small families, but in such large families a
cohesive family network is associated with a greater tendency to
accept the sick role because it is a luxury that the mother can only
enjoy if she has a supportive family. Another important factor
determining whether the patient will consult is the patient's beliefs
about health. For example, the extent to which they believe that
medical care can contribute to the resolution of the particular
problem, or the extent to which they believe that preventive care
can reduce morbidity. Cultural factors may play a large part in
determining these health beliefs.

Perhaps one of the most important factors determining whether
a perceived symptom will lead to a consultation is the patient's
expectations of their doctor. This will largely be determined from
the patient's continuing relationship with the doctor, which will
have been built up over a series of clinical contacts.

It is possible to construct a model that reflects this process of
decision making, which determines when a symptom perceived by
a patient is translated into a consultation with a doctor (Fig. 3.1).
The research that has helped in the understanding of the factors

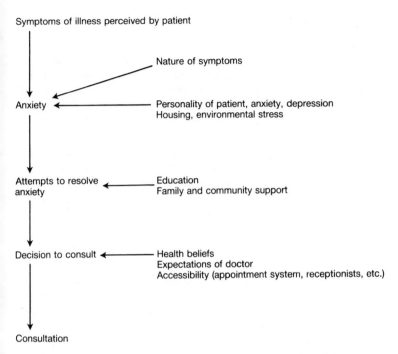

Symptoms of illness perceived by patient

Nature of symptoms

Anxiety ← Personality of patient, anxiety, depression
Housing, environmental stress

Attempts to resolve anxiety ← Education
Family and community support

Decision to consult ← Health beliefs
Expectations of doctor
Accessibility (appointment system, receptionists, etc.)

Consultation

Fig. 3.1.   Factors influencing the decision to consult a doctor.

that influence patients in seeking medical care is important because it helps doctors to understand the demands made on them and to elicit the necessary information to enable them to formulate patients' problems. How relevant is this to the medical student working in general practice and observing the patients seeking care? Some of the calls to the general practitioner might be regarded as unjustifiable by the student, and in some cases, downright unreasonable. Most of them, however, do reflect a cry for help, and the student must become familiar with how to interpret and respond to this cry.

Case 1. Mrs C. called the doctor at 9.00pm on a Saturday because her daughter, Margaret, had severe abdominal pain. By the time the doctor arrived, 1 hour later, Margaret was asleep and the call appeared to be unnecessary. The doctor, however, observed that the child was sharing a bed with three other children. Mr C. had left home and grandma, resplendent in curlers, was surveying the situation critically. It was easy to see why

Mrs C. had felt compelled to call the doctor when the peace of the single room, in which this family was living, had been broken by Margaret's cries of distress.

Case 2. Mrs H. called the doctor at 10.00pm because she had spilt tea on young Georgie and caused a minor burn. The doctor observed that this required a simple dressing. He also observed Mr H. looking decidedly embarrassed. It transpired that he had 'lost his head' at the sight of his son and heir suffering from mild erythema of his chest and had attacked his wife so violently that she had felt compelled to send for the doctor.

Doctors might feel annoyed and students might consider it unreasonable that they are called on to solve what are essentially social problems, but this is almost inevitable in the situation in which they work. It is perhaps easier to just accept these irritations, and to use them as sources of information about the patients in their practice.

Another alarming result of the accessibility of general practitioners is the wide variety of problems about which they are expected to give advice. These reach far beyond the limits of medicine as taught in medical schools. Such subjects as the behaviour of children, adolescence, marriage, and the menopause receive scant attention in the medical curriculum; divorce, house mortgage, and hire purchase debts are normally omitted altogether. Yet general practitioners will be expected to have an opinion about all these problems and many others. Students might feel that doctors are not qualified to deal with such matters and furthermore, that they are outside their terms of service and that it is unreasonable for their patients to make these demands of them. Doctors are no doubt within their rights to adopt such an attitude, but in so doing they should realize that they might be missing some excellent opportunities of gaining insight into the lives of their patients. The knowledge acquired might not be immediately relevant, but in time might prove invaluable in interpreting their patients' responses to stress and disease, and the trust that they will have learned to place in their doctors will greatly facilitate subsequent relationships with them.

Case 3. Mrs F. came to the doctor for advice. Her husband was having an affair with another woman. There was little the doctor could do but he encouraged her to talk about the difficulties in her marriage. The therapeutic value of this consultation was limited, but 6 months later when Mrs F. presented her 4 year old son with enuresis, its diagnostic value became apparent.

Case 4. Mrs D, a very anxious woman of 40, approached the doctor rather diffidently and asked him to talk to her 15 year old son about puberty. The doctor, without enthusiasm, agreed to undertake this task. Three months later, Mrs D. approached the doctor again, deeply distressed. She explained that because he had been so understanding with her son she had gained the confidence to ask him to help her. It transpired that her husband was impotent, a situation that was causing considerable marital stress.

Throughout this book the importance of the knowledge accumulated by general practitioners about their patients is constantly stressed. Much of this is acquired because of the easy access that the patients have to them. This access might lead to unnecessary calls, but by managing such situations with appropriate sympathy or firmness, they will help their patients get to know them and their expectations, and will develop that mutual respect on which harmonious doctor–patient relationships are based. This is something that students can begin to appreciate in a short attachment in general practice.

THE FIELD OF WORK OF THE FAMILY DOCTOR

This is a wide field and when students study general practice they must decide which particular aspects of medicine are important. Perhaps the most satisfactory way of approaching this problem is to look at the population's need for medical care and decide what general practitioners are, by nature of their position, best able to provide and what is more safely or economically administered within the framework of the hospital or social services.

General practitioners are patients' first contact and therefore they must clearly be experts in interpreting the problems presented to them in terms of their patients' needs. This should be regarded as their most important function and therefore prime consideration when identifying priorities in the use of their time. They are ideally situated to provide the continuity of care demanded in the treatment of chronic and incurable disease. Here they will work closely with nursing colleagues who also have the skills and discipline that are necessary to undertake this work. The knowledge that they acquire about their patients and about their environments gives them exceptional advantages in dealing with the problems of personal relationships and psychosocial illness. It also makes them the ideal people to interpret the importance of disease to the individual. The close relationships that they enjoy with their patients provides them with opportunities to educate them about preventive medicine. The development of the primary health care team, consisting of doctor, nurse, and health visitor, is particularly important in this field of primary care.

Hospitals possess different attributes. They contain specialists who, while limited in their breadth of knowledge and in their opportunities for early diagnosis and continuing medical care, have a depth of knowledge that is essential in the investigation and treatment of many diseases. They can provide the supervision and nursing care that are required in serious illness, and they house the staff and equipment that are essential for many modern diagnostic and therapeutic procedures.

These two fields of medicine are distinct but complementary, and in an ideal society should work in perfect harmony. They do however, demand different knowledge and skills, and it is inevitable that when students leave the hsopital they will find it necessary to reorientate their medical thinking to suit their new situation in general practice. Up to this point, students' contact with illness will have been restricted to highly selected groups of patients; selected by general practitioners as needing hospital care. The illnesses will usually have reflected diseases demanding full exam-ination and investigation, which will have led to a diagnosis in most cases. In general practice, however, students meet illness at an early stage in its natural history and despite detailed examina-tion and investigation a precise diagnosis might not be possible at this stage. Many of these illnesses subsequently resolve without treatment. Others develop with time into recognizable entities that justify further investigation. In addition, the student working in general practice will see many patients suffering from chronic diseases in which the diagnosis will have been established many years before and medical care is concerned with the continuing management of the disability that has been produced rather than with intense diagnostic activity.

In their hospital experience, students will have seen patients entering hospital desperately ill and will have enjoyed feelings of success when a correct diagnosis has led to correct treatment and, hopefully, to cure. Not infrequently, however, treatment will have been less successful and patients will then be discharged home. These patients no longer haunt the hospital specialist because they become part of the continuing care provided in general practice, and it is here that students can study the longer term results of in-patient care.

The curative role of the general practitioner may be under-estimated by students, who have become so accustomed to high technology medicine that they fail to appreciate that twenty years ago patients died of pneumonia, developed mastoiditis as a complication of otitis media, required surgery for peptic ulcers, languished in mental hospitals if they suffered from schizophrenia, were admitted to hospital for uncontrolled eczema, and died of malignant hypertension. These life threatening conditions are now the bread and butter of general practice and the doctor's curative role is taken for granted.

Twenty years ago, patients died of poliomyelitis, whooping cough, and measles. Prevention is not dramatic high technology medicine, but the prevention of these disorders in general practice is probably more relevant to public health than that of the expensive medicine that is carried out in hospitals.

When working in general practice students need to adapt to the provision of medical care in the community. This is concerned with the evaluation of early symptoms of illness, most of which reflect self-limiting diseases, and with identifying life-threatening situations within this mass of newly presented symptoms. It is also concerned with efficient and effective treatment of acute infection, with continuing care for chronic disease and disability, and, above all, with effective preventive services.

CONTINUITY OF MEDICAL CARE

General practice presents an unrivalled opportunity for studying the natural history of disease. James Mackenzie, the doyen of general practice, realized this and much of his original work was based on the observation of individuals over a number of years. Many of the earlier pioneers of medicine also advanced medical knowledge by their studies of disease in the community, and in recent years there has been a resurgence of enthusiasm for this type of research.

The accumulation of knowledge about disease, and the ways in which men and women respond to it, is inevitable in general practice, but it can be greatly augmented if doctors make a conscious effort to maintain good records. In this way they can study, for example, the insidious onset of peptic ulceration and chronic bronchitis, the varied responses of hypertension and osteoarthritis to treatment, and the unpredictable course of psoriasis and disseminated sclerosis. The experience thus accrued will influence their history-taking and examination of patients, and will give them a realistic awareness of the probabilities in diagnosis. Above all it will teach them the art of prognosis and help them to anticipate trouble before it occurs.

Apart from the academic or research value of the continuous medical care provided by the general practitioner, it is of great importance to a personal doctor because it implies a continuous relationship over a period of time with his or her patients. Each contact between doctor and patient determines to some extent the relationship that will exist at the next consultation. If the doctor successfully treats one member of the family the others will approach him or her with greater confidence whereas if he or she fails badly in some therapeutic situation their relationship will be adversely affected.

Certain episodes of medical care are of particular value in building up the doctor–patient relationship. The successful treatment of a seriously ill child, successful and fulfilling obstetric medical care, or the sympathetic management of a dying relative, will do more to establish the doctor than many more complex, but less emotionally charged, situations. This can be very noticeable when doctors are faced with chronic incurable disease. If patients have experienced the therapeutic competence of doctors, they will be able to accept the limitations of medical treatment more easily. If their experience in the past has been unfortunate then they might quickly seek a second opinion. The day-to-day management of incurable disease can be difficult. It is humiliating to have to admit defeat. In hospital medicine it is easy to escape by using an unrealistic prognosis or discharging the patient from hospital care, but this avenue is closed to the general practitioner, on whom it would almost certainly rebound.

THE ISOLATION OF THE GENERAL PRACTITIONER

Medical isolation is one of the dangers of general practice. Much of the knowledge acquired after qualifying occurs as a result of discussion between colleagues and this provides a stimulus to make a greater effort. The loss of such discussion is serious because family doctors' work is completely unsupervised and, in the absence of outside criticism, they might begin to lose their own critical faculties. They frequently deal with illness that cannot be easily subjected to a precise diagnosis and they are often called on by their patients to interpret their illnesses in words that they will understand. The illness might be described as a touch of fibrositis or lumbago, or a chill on the liver or kidneys, to make it meaningful or consoling to the patient. It is easy, over the course of years, for doctors to begin to think in these terms without really asking themselves what is going on in the patient's body and mind. There are many people who have been erroneously diagnosed as suffering from prolapsed intervertebral discs, colitis, or migraine, to take but three examples, as a result of the loose thinking that is a constant hazard to the general practitioner.

There appear to be fashions in medical diagnosis that are known not only to doctors but also to laymen, and particularly to that influential body that runs the pharmaceutical industry. Because it is consoling for doctors to make a diagnosis that is amenable to treatment, there is a risk that they will find themselves diagnosing conditions for which treatment is available. The apparent rise in the prevalence of depression in the last two decades might be more closely related to the availability of antidepressant drugs than to any real change in the prevalence of this disorder.

The antidote for this is to take advantage of every opportunity for medical discussion. This is one of the advantages of group practices in which several doctors working together have the chance of comparing notes. About 1000 practices in the United Kingdom have trainee assistants and probably three times this number have medical students attached to them. This provides another important stimulus for doctors to look critically at the care they are providing. It is also one of the main attractions of clinical assistantships in hospitals. General practitioners can reduce their sense of isolation and lack of supervision by establishing close relationships with hospital consultants. Such arrangements serve a dual role. The general practitioners will endeavour to maintain a high standard of medicine for their consultant colleagues and they in turn will try to provide a good hospital service. If this blossoms to the point when both are prepared to give and to accept criticism, it will become even more valuable.

In addition, family doctors can benefit both themselves and their patients by refusing to relinquish all responsibility for the care of their patients when they are admitted to hospital. They should always be prepared to commit themselves to a provisional diagnosis and to follow that patient into the ward and discuss the problem with the consultant. In this way they can often contribute to the correct diagnosis and treatment, will be able to guide the consultant with regard to prognosis, evaluate their own responsibilities in aftercare, and expose themselves to critical discussion. Needless to say, patients are always very reassured to see their own doctor in the hospital ward. The following examples may clarify the advantages of this relationship.

Case 5. Mrs F., aged 30, with four children, developed a swelling in her neck. She was admitted to hospital for a biopsy, which revealed Hodgkins lymphoma. The family doctor visited his patient in hospital and discussed the full implications of her anticipated prolonged period of hospital treatment with the consultant. He made arrangements for the care of her children while she was away, and was able to mobilize the community services to continue her treatment and care after she returned home. This patient's treatment and rehabilitation were directed by mutual discussions between her general practitioner and consultant. The former increased his knowledge of the treatment of lymphoma, and the latter his appreciation of what this entailed for the mother of a young family.

Case 6. Mr M., aged 50, developed malignant hypertension and was admitted to hospital for investigation. This did not reveal any renal cause for his disease, and treatment was started with hypotensive drugs. He was engaged in heavy manual work but his general practitioner was able to arrange a less arduous occupation by consulting with Mr M's employer. He was discharged as soon as reasonable control of his blood pressure had been established and his general practitioner, after discussion with the specialiast, was able to take complete control of Mr M's treatment. He was therefore assured of day-to-day adjustment of his drugs in the environment of his home and work, a more satisfactory arrangement than stabilization of his treatment in the hospital environment. The consultant was thus relieved of a series of out-patient appointments and the general practitioner not only kept abreast of modern hypotensive treatment but also enjoyed taking full responsibility for his patient.

Though general practitioners may, by various means, maintain a high standard of medicine they will soon realize that this is not always the criterion by which their patients will base their assessment of them as family doctors. Many of their greatest medical achievements, such as the early diagnosis of malignant disease will, for obvious reasons, never be known to their patients. They might be surprised at the gratitude that rewards some of their poorest efforts, and the aggression and rancour that might result when they have done their best.

General practice is, of course, much more than a study of the science of medicine. It is a study of life itself and family doctors are often intimately involved with the lives of their patients. In these circumstances it is essential that they should become philosopher as well as doctors. They must develop a philosophy of life that allows them to detach themselves from the common emotional crises that surround them and to view life and death, and success and failure, in perspective. It is helpful to accept a philosophy that does not directly relate the efforts indulged in life to the rewards received, although the emotional rewards in general practice are very considerable.

REFERENCES

Dunnell, K., and Carwright, A. (1972). *Medicine takers, prescribers, and hoarders*. Routledge and Kegan Paul, London.

Morrell, D. and Wale, C. (1976). Symptoms perceived and recorded by patients. *Journal of the Royal College of General Practitioners*, **26,** 398–403.

4

Solving problems in general practice

In medical education, the term 'diagnosis' has often been used in the rather restricted way that is defined in the Concise Oxford Dictionary, 'Identification of disease by means of patients symptoms, etc.'. Limiting the term diagnosis to describing the process by which disease is identified, does not recognize what usually occurs in the general practitioner's consulting room. Here the patient presents one or more symptoms, which leads to a dialogue between patient and doctor from which the main problems that the patient is experiencing are identified. Sometimes these problems are further clarified by physical examination and investigation, then a programme of management is agreed. To avoid semantic difficulties, the term 'problem solving' has sometimes been used to replace the term diagnosis to emphasize that the explanation of the symptoms presented might not necessarily be solved by the diagnosis of a disease in terms of pathological changes in the body, but might be solved because of a variety of other factors. An alternative approach to this difficulty is to emphasize that diagnosis should not be restricted to the interpretation of symptoms in terms of disease, but should be expressed in terms of physical, social, and psychological factors. In this book the term diagnosis will be used in this broad sense.

Diagnosis in general practice is therefore concerned with the whole situation that the individual is experiencing when he develops symptoms of illness or incapacity that interfere with life or cause anxiety sufficient to lead to a medical consultation. Many symptoms prsented are mild or self-limiting, or are due to infections or minor trauma. Others reflect personal or social problems leading to incapacity, and a few reflect a serious pathological process, which if treated inappropriately may lead to serious illness or death. The first stage in the general practitioner's approach to new symptoms of illness must therefore be to identify those problems that carry with them a serious threat to health. This diagnostic approach must be concerned with confirming or eliminating the possibility of serious disease. In situations in which serious disease is present, such as appendicitis, pneumonia, or myocardial infarction, the immediate management response will be a major therapeutic intervention either in the community or by referral to a specialist. In many cases there will be no obvious major pathology and the doctor will be faced with the problem of evaluating the symptoms in terms of the psychological or social factors that might be influencing this new request for medical care.

THE DIAGNOSTIC MODEL IN GENERAL PRACTICE

Inductive reasoning

Medical students will, when they join their general practice clerkship, have experience of a diagnostic process that is often described as inductive reasoning. They will have been taught how to collect information from patients about their presenting complaint and, by a 'systems review', to identify any other important symptoms. They will also have learned how to take a family and social history, but with little understanding of the value of this to the patient's presenting symptoms. They will have learned how to carry out a full physical examination and how to carry out certain routine investigations. All the information thus collected is then brought together to reach a diagnosis. This is a practical way of teaching medical students to learn the skills of history taking and clinical examination, but it does not reflect the real diagnostic model that is used either in hospital or in general practice. It is in general practice clerkships that the inappropriateness of this diagnostic model is most likely to cause medical students serious problems. Here they will see that such a model is inappropriate when sorting out the primary demands for medical care initiated by patients at an early stage in the natural history of illness. It might be that during their general practice clerkships, they realize for the first time that the surgeon and physician in the out-patient department also use a very different diagnostic model.

The hypothetico-deductive method

The diagnostic model that is often used in real life situations in both hospital and general practice has been described as a hypothetico-deductive model. In response to patients' symptoms, doctors, at an early stage during interview, form a diagnostic hypothesis. They then test this hypothesis by asking appropriate questions and by examining or investigating the patients. If the hypothesis is sustained, they then develop a plan of management. It must be stressed that at this stage they might or might not have made a diagnosis in terms of a specific disease. If further enquiries fail to sustain the original hypothesis, they return to 'go' and develop an alternative one. In practise, the process might not be as clear cut as this description suggests, and more than one hypothesis might be entertained at a fairly early stage in the interview.

Case 7. Pamela P, aged 20, presented with right sided abdominal pain, which had been present for 24 hours. It was a constant pain that had disturbed her sleep the previous night. She had noticed mild nausea and some increase in frequency of micturition. The initial hypothesis concerned the possiblity of appendicitis or a urinary tract infection. Examination showed a mild pyrexia and tachycardia thus supporting the hypothesis of infection. Abdominal examination showed tenderness low in the right iliac fossa and urinalysis showed no proteinuria. The hypothesis was then altered to consider pelvic inflammatory disease and further questioning disclosed that Pamela had noticed some vaginal discharge and pain on sexual intercourse. She had a marked tenderness to the right and pain on moving the cervix on pelvic examination. There was also a profuse smelly vaginal discharge that was swabbed and sent to the laboratory for culture. Treatment was instituted with metronidazole and tetracycline and the symptoms and signs rapidly resolved thus confirming the diagnosis.

Pattern recognition

Very often doctors working in general practice make diagnoses on the basis of their previous experiences. They will have seen most illnesses before and immediately recognize them again. Examples include conditions such as inguinal hernia, herpes zoster, and rodent ulcer. The intellectual activity devoted to decision making in such cases is minimal. Pattern recognition does, however, depend on a period of exposure to the common diseases presenting in general practice. Experienced doctors might have little difficulty in immediately recognizing scabies, pityriasis rosea, hayfever, polymyalgia rheumatica, or tennis elbow, but medical students might be somewhat confused by this diagnostic approach. The next case presents an example.

Case 8. Nicholas R., aged 5, was brought to the trainee doctor with a rash. The trainee had seen the child 24 hours earlier with an apparent upper respiratory infection and had prescribed penicillin. When the child consulted again, the trainee suspected that this was an allergic reaction to the penicillin. He consulted his trainer who immediately recognized measles. The trainer had seen numerous 'measley' children; miserable, pyrexial, with an irritable cough, and a very characteristic rash. The trainee had tried to take an intellectual approach to solving the problems of this child, while the trainer made an instant diagnosis.

Use of knowledge and information in diagnosis

The diagnostic models that have been presented suggest that clinicians collect information from patients by history taking, examination, and investigation and that this information is then matched against their knowledge base. It might therefore be expected that doctors who have greater communication skills in terms of history taking and examination, and who have a greater knowledge base, might be better diagnosticians. There is some evidence that this is not so, and that knowledge is stored in terms of its relevance to the clinical situations commonly encountered. The potential for interpretation of an array of clinical information is vast and it is hardly surprising that much practice is needed to arrange the memory structures in the brain appropriately to deal with the problems frequently encountered. Doctors working in a specialty appear to store knowledge selectively in their memories and can respond to characteristics of the particular disorders common to that specialty. General practitioners probably also selectively store information that is of importance to them in their day-to-day care of patients.

THE DIAGNOSTIC PROCESS IN GENERAL PRACTICE

New symptoms of illness presented in general practice might reflect: serious life threatening disease; appropriate or inappropriate anxiety; minor self-limiting disease; major or minor psychological and social problems. In many cases the physical, social, and psychological elements interact in determining when the patient decides to present problems to the doctor. It is sometimes helpful to consider the diagnostic process in four stages.

Stage I—Is there major pathology, physical, mental, or social, that has provoked this patient to consult?

Stage II—Why has this patient presented this problem at this particular time?

Stage III—What is the significance of this problem or disease to this particular patient?

Stage IV—Is there any other factor that is important in the management of this patient's problem?

Stage I—Is there major pathology, physical, mental, or social, that has provoked this patient to consult?

The first stage in the diagnostic process is concerned with the general practitioner's vital role in identifying serious life threatening disease at an early stage and responding appropriately to hopefully prevent serious morbidity. Examples of such conditions include appendicitis, pneumonia, myocardial infarction, and ectopic pregnancy. In practice this is not an easy task because patients complaining of chest or abdominal pain, cough, tiredness, or shortness of breath present every day, and the probability in general practice of any one of these symptoms being caused by serious life threatening disease is very small.

Stage II—Why has this patient presented this problem at this particular time?

Having excluded serious pathology the general practitioner is then faced with a wide variety of symptoms that might reflect either minor self-limiting disease or the very early stages of something more serious. Attempting to explain the patient's problems in terms of disease often fails to help understand the patient's real problem. The general practitioner must therefore delve deeper into different areas of human behaviour and in doing so will become aware of the factors influencing demand for medical care described in Chapter 3, and will try to find out from the patient what has produced this particular consultation.

Stage III—What is the significance of the problem or disease to this particular patient?

This stage attempts to relate the current problem to the patient as a whole. For example a skin infection in a diabetic, influenza in a chronic bronchitic, or a urinary tract infection in a patient with multiple sclerosis. Each of these diagnoses has a special significance.

Stage IV—Is there any other factor present that is important in managing this patient's problem?

This often embraces social and environmental problems. The single parent with dependent children who cannot afford to be ill; the self-employed 'bread-winner' has special problems if he develops a disabling disease; the elderly carer for a disabled spouse encounters special difficulties. Some examples might help to explain the diagnostic approach to such problems.

Case 9. Mrs L. was a 30-year-old housewife complaining of headache, shivering, and aching limbs, of sudden onset. A diagnosis of influenza was made (stage I), occurring in the middle of an epidemic (stage II). She had a history of chest trouble following upper respiratory infections due to kyphoscoliosis of the spine and poor chest expansion (stage III). Her husband was a salesman working away from home during the week and she had two children of school age (stage IV). In this relatively simple illness, the full diagnosis showed many problems, the recognition of which were essential before complete treatment of this patient could be instituted.

Case 10. Mr H., aged 49, complained of shortness of breath on exertion. History and examination led to a diagnosis of chronic bronchitis (stage I). The recent foggy weather had caused an exacerbation of his symptoms and prompted the consultation (stage II). He worked on the railways, cycling to and from work, and found this increasingly difficult. He was also finding that the cold nights made his chest worse when he was on night shift (stage III). He had four children at school and could not afford to change his job. His father died of cor-pulmonale (stage IV).

Case 11. An urgent call was made on a Saturday afternoon for Mrs T., aged 32, who was reported to have collapsed. After taking a history, a confident diagnosis of over-breathing was made (stage I). Examination showed no abnormality, except for the presence of cardiac extra-systoles. She recounted that she had suffered from heart trouble all her life and that, on occasions, she collapsed in this way. Further history taking disclosed that the present attack had been brought on by her husband threatening to walk out on her (stage II). It then transpired that she had been told that she must never have children because of her heart. She had always found sexual intercourse unattractive and, because of her heart-trouble, her husband had been persuaded to forego his marital rights and therefore sought satisfaction elsewhere (stages III and IV). A cardiologist subsequently confirmed the absence of any cardiac abnormality, but a complete cure of the iatrogenic heart disease and its complications proved more difficult.

Case 12. Mrs S., aged 36, complained of tiredness, palpitations, and shortness of breath on exertion. The first stage diagnosis was anaemia due to menorrhagia, but correction of this did not cure her symptoms. Further enquiry disclosed that Mrs S. had been married at the age of 26, eight years before her first baby was born. Her husband did not want a baby because he felt that it disrupted his social life and interfered with his prospects in business. Mrs S. had satisfied her maternal instincts, but at the expense of marital harmony.

This diagnostic approach should not, of course, be peculiar to general practice. It is equally applicable in the hospital. The difference in approach is due not only to the knowledge normally available to the family doctor but also to the results of treatment as they affect the practitioners concerned. For doctors in hospital, stage I diagnoses might suffice. In this artificial environment they will treat the obvious pathological conditions and then discharge patients as cured. As far as they are concerned, this is the end of the story. If general practitioners fail to elucidate the true problems, they will fail to produce complete cures, and patients whom they feel should be restored to health, will continue to attend their surgeries. There is then a risk that doctors will label these patients as neurotic, or send them to the nearest hospital to get rid of them. Patients are thus penalized for doctors' diagnostic errors and situations are created that are very difficult to rectify.

The continuity of medical care characteristic of general practice renders every consultation of great importance to both doctors and patients. Doctors' success or failure on these occasions will influence their future relationships with their patients. To the patients, accurate interpretation is probably less important than a sympathetic appreciation of the complete problem. It is uncommon for patients to think any less of doctors because they admit that they cannot solve certain clinical problems and need specialist advice, but they will quickly lose faith if they feel that doctors are either not interested or are unable to appreciate why they as patients are so concerned.

The demands of patients for a satisfactory explanation of their diseases will often place doctors in a position in which the needs of their patients will be in apparent conflict with their scientific concepts. This is a feature of general practice, which may, with time, endanger the intellectual honesty of doctors. At the present stage of education of the public in medical matters, an answer is expected to the question 'What is the matter, doctor?' The answer is expected to be in terms that convey something to the patient, which means that the disease must be fitted into a small catalogue of acceptable diseases. This catalogue is not published, but includes the common childhood complaints, which have become household words, and those medical conditions currently appearing in the daily press and in various homely magazines.

The fact that a precise diagnosis cannot be given for about 50 per cent of the illnesses seen in general practice is not yet appreciated by the general public. This places general practitioners in a quandary. If they wish to be scientifically accurate, they will have to express their diagnostic ignorance. Though such honesty is praiseworthy in the privacy of their own minds, it deprives patients of the comfort that they need, and will often impair the efficiency of treatment. There are occasions when doctors can explain that they are treating the symptoms rather than the disease, and that the final outcome will justify this approach. There are other occasions, however, when they must be concerned about the patient's peace of mind.

Case 13. The doctor was called late at night to see John N., aged 4. He had a high fever, the cause of which was not apparent on examination. His parents were seriously alarmed by this fever, which had come on suddenly and had made John delirious. They wanted to know the reason—they wanted a diagnosis. These parents were not very intelligent. The doctor had to decide, in the few seconds available, whether they could accept an explanation of the situation, or whether they would be more comforted by a speculative diagnosis. He felt certain that the child was suffering from an acute infection, the site of which not yet being apparent. He advised symptomatic treatment, which quickly brought the child's temperature down and, to satisfy the parents' enquiry, explained that the child had an acute pharyngitis. Parents and child slept well. In the morning signs of otitis media were present and treatment was instituted accordingly.

In this case, the doctor could not make a scientifically accurate stage I diagnosis and so he proceeded with stages III and IV and treated these, to the best of his ability, by explaining in words acceptable to the parents. He could have said 'John clearly has an infection, but I do not know what it is. I am sure that it is nothing serious, and we will wait for the physical signs to develop before instituting specific treatment'. He would no doubt have said this to some parents, but in the case in question this would have only further alarmed the parents and so he took the more humane approach.

In dealing with an unknown diagnosis, the first consideration must be the safety of the patient. If the symptom could indicate a potentially lethal condition such as appendicitis, meningitis, or a coronary thrombosis, then prevarication is inadmissible and a domiciliary consultation or hospital admission must be arranged. A vast amount of illness is, however, presented to the family doctor at such an early stage that a definitive diagnosis is not possible, and the patient is quite clearly not going to be endangered by a policy of waiting. In this case, the doctor's immediate task is to deal, not so much with the pathological problem, but with the whole situation. This will often mean symptomatic treatment of the patient, but above all sympathetic management of the family in terms of an explanation that can be comprehended by the relatives. This might require the use of unscientific and essentially vague language, but if such is necessary to comfort the individuals concerned and to clarify the situation for them, it is amply justified. An attempt is often made to separate psychiatric illness from physical disease. Surveys have shown a ninefold difference between doctors in the frequency of diagnosis of mental illness. Fifty-one per cent of the variation could be accounted for by ecological and observer factors. Body and mind are parts of each individual and anything affecting one will inevitably affect the other. In the diagnostic field, over-simplification is highly dangerous, and the diagnosis of neurosis often indicates the inability of the doctor to understand the impact of some physical abnormality on an unstable personality. To ignore the body and concentrate exclusively on the mind might cause as much suffering as the reverse process of treating the body as a depersonalized object of scientific enquiry.

It is this interdependence of body and mind that makes diagnosis in psychosomatic disorders so difficult. In recent years great emphasis has been placed on the importance of mental ill health in the production of physical symptoms. Some have suggested that all general practitioners should have experience of superficial psychoanalysis, and far more facilities should be introduced for deep psychoanalysis by experts in this field. While the protagonists of this approach have done a great deal for general practice in elucidating, or at least highlighting, the complexities of the doctor–patient relationship, the extremists have introduced some concepts that are dangerous. Very few people could be submitted to psychoanalysis without unearthing some fact from their past that has unpleasant associations and was a potential source of mental or bodily disease. It is the next step, often hastily taken, which immediately attributes this association to the present symptom complex, that can be so misguided. It is easy to attribute every symptom, which cannot be interpreted on physical grounds, to a psychiatric disorder. A patient with pain in the neck might be shown to have cervical spondylosis, but this does not mean that a cause and effect are necessarily established because many people over the age of 50 have cervical spondylosis. Equally, a person with a pain in the neck might have an unsatisfactory sex life, but this is just as likely to be incidental as causative.

Case 14. Mrs M. had a 3-year history of upper abdominal pains that were not typical of any pathological entity. Barium meal was normal. She had a very unhappy married life with a husband who was often out of work and was in constant financial difficulty. Questions about her early life disclosed much deprivation and hardship. It was concluded that this was the cause of her symptoms. She had requested frequent calls to her home, but having once been labelled as suffering from anxiety, she received little sympathy from her medical attendants. The doctor was suddenly shaken from his apathy by her complaint of pain radiating through to the right scapular region. Cholecystogram showed a gall-bladder full of stones, and surgical treatment provided complete relief of her symptoms. Now, despite her family difficulties, she has a happy life and rarely calls the doctor.

The opposite state of affairs occurs just as often.

Case 15. Mr S. had a history of peptic ulceration, confirmed 2 years previously by barium meal. This was treated successfully and for a year he was symptom-free. He returned to the doctor complaining that 'My ulcer is troubling me again'. He was treated with cimetidine, but with only partial relief, and became a frequent surgery attender. In desperation the doctor referred him to a surgeon to be considered for operative treatment. Fortunately, the surgeon proved to be a more complete doctor than the general practitioner and was able to elicit that Mr S. was in the midst of serious personal problems, which he had not been able to discuss with his family doctor. It was also pointed out that Mr S.'s symptoms were no longer typical of peptic ulceration. The doctor had, in fact, accepted the patient's diagnosis without question and had failed to identify the real problem.

Both these cases illustrate the danger of labelling a patient with a diagnosis and of forgetting that life is dynamic, and that what holds good today might be false a few years later. General practitioners, who are exposed to their patients for many years, are at a greater risk of labelling in this way than their specialist colleagues. Certain diagnostic labels are particularly dangerous. 'I'm getting a lot of migraine' might mean anything from a cerebral tumour to depression. 'A touch of indigestion' often covers myocardial ischaemia, and 'my bronchitis' might indicate a carcinoma of the lung.

Case 16. Mr H. had suffered from chronic bronchitis for years. During one winter he became progressively more breathless on exertion. Treatment was directed to his bronchitis. After several weeks he confided that he was waking in the night with attacks of acute dyspnoea, and it was only then that it was noticed that he had become severely hypertensive.

If doctors are to provide continuous medical care for their patients, they must be prepared to review their diagnoses constantly. This is particularly important in the case of the chronically sick and the elderly, and it is good to regularly provide time to make fresh approaches to them and see if any new features have appeared in their illnesses that demand modifications of treatment. It is surprising how often such reviews open up new avenues for therapeutic endeavours, and it also reassures patients that they have not been thrown to one side as hopeless cases. Some general practitioners have adopted the practise of introducing flow charts into the medical records of patients suffering from chronic diseases such as diabetes, congestive cardiac failure, hypertension, and epilepsy (Fig. 4.1). They review their patients' progress annually

IDEAL WT. _____ DIET ⟨ Cals. _____ 　　　 Gms.　CBH	NAME _____ DIABETES REVIEW FLOW SHEET					
DATE						
SYMPTOMS	RIGHT	LEFT	RIGHT	LEFT	RIGHT	LEFT
VISUAL ACUITY						
CATARACT						
FUNDAL CHANGES — DOTS						
FUNDAL CHANGES — BLOTS						
FUNDAL CHANGES — NEW VESSELS						
FUNDAL CHANGES — EXUDATES						
PULSES — POST. TIB.						
PULSES — D. PEDIS						
ANKLE JERKS						
VIBRATION SENSE						
FINE TOUCH						
URINE — GLUCOSE						
URINE — PROTEIN						
URINE — BLOOD						
BLOOD — GLUCOSE						
BLOOD — UREA						
BLOOD PRESSURE						
WEIGHT (KGS.)						
HOME URINE TESTING						
DRUG THERAPY						
ASSESSMENT						
PLAN						

Fig. 4.1. An example of a flow chart for diabetes.

and, by recording this systematically, can easily recognize any major changes and, if necessary, review their diagnoses.

One of the great problems facing students in general practice is to assess the diagnostic significance of certain symptoms. They will have been brought up to deal with the highly selected group of patients seen in hospital in which the significance of a certain presenting symptom might be quite different from that of the same symptom brought to the general practitioner. The patient arriving in hospital with abdominal pain or cough is likely to be suffering from some demonstrable pathology, but in general practice the probability of this is far lower. The initial reaction is to diagnose serious disease more often than it exists, and only time and experience will enable students to develop a more balanced outlook. There is a risk, however, that familiarity with minor illness might lead to the opposite extreme occurring. Thus from assuming the worst until proved otherwise, doctors might find themselves lulled into a false security until they are roused from it by some unfortunate misdiagnosis.

In coping with this problem, students in general practice should study the incidence of different diseases at the primary care level. In addition, it is important to remember that practices vary considerably in the basic characteristics of the population of which they are comprised. In a practice in any of the slum areas of our big cities an itchy rash would immediately raise the possibility of scabies whereas in a practice in a middle class area this would come well down the diagnostic list. Similarly, a common symptom such as cough might have a different significance in a practice in an industrial area in Lancashire from that in a practice on a housing estate in Sussex. It is therefore necessary to study not only the morbidity in general practice at large but also the morbidity within a particular population. In some places the local idiom might present symptoms peculiar to the area. In Scotland, a child might be 'felled' or 'aye greetin'. In parts of England young ladies tend to be 'run down' and men 'under the weather'.

In interpreting the symptoms presented, knowledge is required of two separate yet related aspects of illness in the community. The first is concerned with the interpretation of the symptoms presented at the primary care level, and the second with understanding which patients perceiving symptoms consult the doctor. The latter has been considered in some detail in Chapter 3.

Consideration of the diagnostic probabilities in response to symptoms in general practice remains to be discussed in this chapter.

DIAGNOSTIC PROBABILITIES IN GENERAL PRACTICE

The probability of a particular symptom leading to a particular diagnosis is very different in general practice compared with that in hospital practice. Standard medical textbooks, however, are usually based on hospital practice and are written by doctors with hospital experience only. Students in general practice must therefore review their knowledge in the light of the situation in which they are working.

In 1972 I described the fourteen symptoms most commonly presented in my practice over a period of one year. During this time 5325 new symptoms were presented by 3500 patients. The diagnoses recorded in response to these symptoms were analysed (Appendix 1). The doctors taking part in this study were in no way constrained to reach a diagnosis in pathological terms and if no diagnosis could be made they simply recorded the symptom in the diagnostic box. In addition, the diagnosis recorded did not necessarily reflect the real reason for the consultation in terms of the patient's problems. The results of the study, based on the doctors' immediate responses to new symptoms, clearly indicated that most of the symptoms were attributed to common, self-limiting, non-life threatening diseases. With some symptoms, for example disturbance of bowel and gastric function, no definite diagnosis was made in a large proportion of cases. Only the most common diagnoses are included in the tables, and the group 'others' contains a variety of diagnoses that occurred infrequently. The size of this group gives some idea of the range of diagnoses recorded, varying from 10 per cent of the patients presenting with a cough to nearly 30 per cent of those presenting with a headache.

The rarity of some of the classical diagnoses, for example coronary thrombosis in patients presenting with chest pain and appendicitis in patients presenting with abdominal pain, will be noted compared with the relative frequency with which sprains, strains, and trauma of various sorts were held responsible for these symptoms. Psychiatric diagnoses were infrequently recorded by the doctors.

This does not necessarily imply that a psychiatric illness was not responsible for the symptom. It might simply mean that the doctors were disinclined to label new symptoms with a psychiatric diagnosis at the first consultation. This exercise suggests that the standard textbooks on differential diagnosis cannot be applied to the diagnostic situation in general practice. The textbook 'Practice' published by Longmans and written entirely by general practitioners, gives a detailed description of the diagnostic probabilities of common symptoms presented in general practice (Cormack J., *et al.* 1987).

EARLY DIAGNOSIS

One of the most important tasks of the general practitioner is the early diagnosis of serious disease. The difficulties involved in the evaluation of minor illness have already been mentioned, and it was pointed out that the doctor is often expected to make a diagnosis before the pathognomonic signs have made their appearances. This also applies in more serious illnesses, such as pneumonia, when making the diagnosis at an early stage might depend on recognizing the significance of an altered respiratory rate rather than recognizing all the altered physical signs described in the textbook. Though early diagnosis is important, sequences of events are usually such that, even if doctors miss the early signs, illnesses will quickly develop and reveal themselves. As long as doctors remain accessible to their patients they will nearly always be given a second chance. It is more difficult, yet more important, to recognize the early variations from normal that herald the onset of neoplastic, degenerative, mental disease, or endocrine imbalance. It is necessary to study those factors that promote the correct interpretation of the earliest symptoms of disease.

Early diagnosis initially depends on the patient. He or she must approach the doctor with a complaint. This first approach might be delayed for a variety of reasons, of which the commonest is probably fear. Though fear of the diagnosis might be a potent factor, fear of the doctor might be equally as important. Some patients with trivial complaints constantly attend doctors and it is very easy for these doctors to develop a negative approach to such patients and miss the one symptom that is significant. Others visit doctors only when they are seriously ill. One of the great arts of general practice is to teach the patients how to use doctors in a rational manner. The first step in achieving this is the establishment of a mutual understanding so that patients know that they can approach doctors easily, confident that they will be taken seriously. If they fear that doctors will not be interested, they might be tempted to embellish their symptoms, or behave aggressively in the hope of attracting attention. Doctors must resist any temptation to dismiss symptoms that might be a source of anxiety to the patient, even if they are trivial. It must be remembered that patients usually have a preconceived idea of the significance of their complaint, and however inaccurate this might be, any suggestion of ridicule will do untold damage.

Once patients realize that they can discuss any problem with their doctor and receive a sympathetic response, their approach will usually become more direct. This not only saves time, but also avoids much irritation. As doctors establish their position of trust, they soon find that they can provide guidance, and even admonition, which will be accepted. Gradually mutual respect develops and in these circumstances, troublesome patients and difficult doctors cease to exist.

Naturally there are some patients and some doctors who are too suspicious or obstinate ever to develop such a relationship, and no doubt every general practitioner can think of occasions when such a relationship was impossible. Insecure patients might find it impossible to trust anybody, including their doctors and might behave aggressively. The radio and press often exaggerate the ability of the medical profession to cure disease and doctors' impotence in the face of chronic disease might be interpreted by patients as incompetence. The news media tend to over-emphasize the science of medicine, with its dramatic appeal, without recognizing its limitations. Science makes a great contribution to medicine and to early diagnosis, but before the diagnostic machine is set in motion, individuals have to complain of some perceived abnormality in the structure or function of their body and this complaint must be assessed. It is the ease of the relationship between doctor and patient that determines the stage at which this complaint will be presented and the subsequent action taken. It is on this relationship, more than on any other factor, that early diagnosis depends.

Doctors' assessment of patients' presenting symptoms is the

next stage in the process of early diagnosis. This part of the proceedings cannot be divorced from their relationship with patients, because it depends very largely on their knowledge of the individuals concerned. This will be supplemented by good medical records, which can be a mine of information. They will show how often patients have consulted their doctors, the sort of problems for which they considered it necessary to invoke medical aid, and their response to ill health and the various stresses of life. Experienced general practitioners will assess these facts with scarcely a conscious effort, but students will have to analyse them and try to build up pictures of the type of people with whom they are dealing.

The medical records currently used in general practice in the United Kingdom were developed nearly half a century ago. They are totally inadequate to store the information needed for decision-making in general practice. In the United Kingdom and throughout the world a great deal of work is being undertaken to devise a satisfactory record. The problem orientated approach is being widely adopted. The essential characteristic of this is that it displays the main problems experienced by the patient, so that every new problem can be reviewed against the background of the patient's previous experiences. New problems are expressed in terms of the patient's complaint and the objective findings, assessment of the situation, and plan of action. This is illustrated in Fig. 4.2.

In general practice, the need to highlight significant long term problems must be balanced against the need to record every problem encountered. To overcome this difficulty, it is necessary to define those problems that merit inclusion in a summary problem list. These may be defined as those problems that are important for doctors to be aware of in providing continuing care for their patients. By prominently displaying such problems in the medical record, doctors may be alerted to respond appropriately to patients' presenting symptoms thus promoting early diagnosis (Fig. 4.3).

Knowledge plays a part in the final stage of early symptomatic diagnosis, but this knowledge—the knowledge of medicine—is common to all doctors. Certain symptoms are well recognized as heralding the onset of serious disease, for example weightloss, intermenstrual bleeding, sleep disturbance, or a sudden change in bowel habit. General practitioners should be alive to these

Date	S/V O	½	CONSULTATION DATA	PROBLEM	No.
			OCCUPATION Taxi Driver		
			MARITAL STATUS Married		
2/4/86	S	2	S- Symptom free	DIABETES	1
			O Home test. Blood sugars 7-11	MELLITUS	
			BP 170/100 Fundi ✓ Pulses ✓ Urine ✓	Hypertension	2
			P R/ Atanolol 100mg Daily		
			Insulatard 20U. AM		
			16U. PM		
3/7/86	S	1	S- Rash on hands Decorating bedroom	Contact	3
			O - Eczematous rash on hands and wrists	Eczema	
			P - Advice		
			R/ 1% Hydrocortisone Cream		
4/10/86	S	2	P. R/ Influvac	Immunisation	1
8/12/86	S	1	S- Cough, fever, yellow spit, breathless		
			O - T 37	Ac BRONCHITIS	4
			Chest-Prolonged Expiration widespread rôles & rhones		
			BP 160/100 Blood sugars 10-14		
			P R/ Amoxycillin 250mg +ds cc.		

Fig. 4.2. Problem orientated record card.

	Date		PROBLEM	ACTION
	1979	1	THYROTOXICOSIS 131	Annual Thyroid Function
	1981	2	HYSTERECTOMY (Fibroids)	
	1983	3	HYPERTENSION	See flowchart.
	1985	4	PENICILLIN ALLERGY	
	1986	5	PERNICIOUS ANAEMIA	Annual Blood Count

Fig. 4.3. An example of a typical summary record card listing a patient's problems.

significant symptoms and should become experts in picking them out from the many mundane symptoms with which they are presented. Occasionally the vital symptom is presented, not by the patient, but by a relative or friend. This may take several forms. A husband or wife might come direct to the doctor to express anxiety about the health of their partner. Alternatively, they themselves might present with some trivial complaint to discuss their anxiety about another member of the family. Sometimes the children might be brought to start a consultation that will provide an opportunity for the parent to discuss his or her fears. These are situations with which doctors must become familiar if they are to take full advantage of them.

Finally, once doctors' suspicions are aroused they must have the organization and facilities for examining and investigating patients in whom they suspect early disease. This will be discussed in later chapters. Although essential if doctors are to enjoy the full satisfaction of this vital role in their work, it is, in some ways, the least important stage in the process of early symptomatic diagnosis.

This chapter has been concerned with the knowledge and skills needed by doctors to identify the problems presented in general practice and the ways in which information, derived from history taking and examination, is integrated to reach a diagnosis. The next two chapters are concerned with acquiring communication skills and with the application of clinical skills in contributing to the diagnostic process in general practice.

REFERENCES

Morrell, D. (1972). Symptom interpretation in general practice. *Journal of the Royal College of General Practitioners,* **22,** 297–309.

Cormack, J., Marinker, M., and Morrell, D. (1987). *'Practice': clinical management in general practice.* Longmans, London.

APPENDIX

This appendix describes the diagnoses recorded by three doctors in response to 5325 consultations at which new symptoms were presented. A new symptom was defined as a symptom that the patient had not presented to any doctor in the preceding year. I reported this study in 1972.

1. Cough

This was the commonest symptom and was recorded on 527 occasions. The highest rate was recorded in the age group 0 to 4 years, and the rate in this age group was twice that recorded in any other. The rate for males was higher than for females under the age of 15 years, but thereafter higher rates were recorded in females. Analysis by social class showed the highest rates in social class III and the lowest in social classes I and II. The diagnoses recorded were:

Diagnosis	Number of consultations
Acute bronchitis	190
Common cold	185
Influenza	35
Chronic bronchitis	33
Laryngitis and tracheitis	31
Pneumonia	10
Whooping cough	4
Others	39
Total	527

2. Rashes

A rash was the complaint at 302 consultations (165 females; 137 males; ratio = 1.2:1.0). The rate recorded for children under the age of 5 years was nearly double that in any other age group. The rate for females aged 5–24 years was higher than for males, but thereafter there was little sex difference. Analysis by social class showed the highest rates in social class III. The diagnoses recorded were:

Diagnosis	Number of consultations
Allergic dermatoses	46
Rubella	44
Dermatitis including contact dermatitis	42
Eczema	39
Dermatophytosis	12
Herpes zoster	11
Psoriasis	10
Scarlet fever	9
Impetigo	8
Chickenpox	7
Acne	6
Others	68
Total	302

3. Sore throat

This symptom was recorded on 287 occasions (162 females; 125 males). The highest rate was recorded in females aged 15–24 years, followed by girls aged 5–14 and males in the same age group. There was little social class difference in the presentation of this symptom. The diagnoses recorded were:

Diagnosis	Number of consultations
Tonsillitis	212
Common cold	32
Laryngitis and tracheitis	12
Influenza	8
Psychiatric disorders	5
Others	18
Total	287

4. Abdominal pain

This symptom was recorded on 197 occasions (104 females; 93 males). The highest rates were recorded in boys and girls aged

5–14 years, but this symptom was one of the most evenly distributed through the age groups and between social classes. The diagnoses recorded were:

Diagnosis	Number of consultations
Colic	36
Sprains and strains	22
Peptic ulcer	15
Disorders of gastric function	15
Other disease of intestines and peritoneum	15
Other disease of stomach and duodenum	13
Psychiatric disorders	14
Appendicitis	8
Pyelonephritis and cystitis	8
Tonsillitis	3
Malignant neoplasms	2
Others	46
Total	197

5. Disturbances of bowel function

This symptom was recorded at 187 consultations (94 females; 93 males). The highest rates were recorded in children under the age of 5 years. Apart from this age group, the symptom was evenly distributed between age groups, males and females, and social classes. The diagnoses recorded were:

Diagnosis	Number of consultations
Symptomatic diagnosis (diarrhoea)	80
Symptomatic diagnosis (constipation)	12
Other diseases of the intestine and peritoneum	55
Psychiatric disorders	4
Others	56
Total	207

6. Spots, sores, and ulcers

This group of symptoms was recorded at 182 consultations (103 females; 79 males). The highest rates were recorded in both sexes between the ages of 5 and 14 years. Between 15 and 44 years much higher rates were recorded for females than males. This group of symptoms was very rare over the age of 65 years. The diagnoses recorded were:

Diagnosis	Number of consultations
Impetigo	26
Boil or carbuncle	21
Disease of sweat or sebaceous glands	21
Lacerations	15
Chickenpox	13
Warts	12
Others	74
Total	182

7. Back pain

This symptom was recorded on 172 occasions (90 females; 82 males). It was uncommon under the age of 25 years and the highest rates were recorded in both males and females between 45 and 64 years. Apart from 'cough' it was the commonest symptom in patients aged over 65 years. It was most often seen in social class III; lowest rates were recorded in social classes I and II. The diagnoses recorded were:

Diagnosis	Number of consultations
Sprains	74
Fibrositis and muscular rheumatism	35
Prolapsed intervertebral disc	14
Lumbago	9
Superficial injuries and contusions	7
Osteoarthritis	4
Psychiatric disorders	4
Others	3
	26
Total	172

8. Chest pain

This symptom was recorded at 168 consultations (85 females; 83 males). It was rare under the age of 15 years and the highest rates were recorded in the age group 45–64 years with little difference between the sexes. There was no difference in the rates between the social classes. The diagnoses recorded were:

Diagnosis	Number of consultations
Fibrositis and muscular rheumatism	26
Sprains and strains	19
Psychiatric disorders	14
Pleurisy	13
Acute bronchitis	12
Diseases of the buccal activity and oesophagus	11
Contusions and superficial abrasions	9
Laryngitis and tracheitis	7
Pneumonia	7
Coronary thrombosis	5
Others	45
Total	168

9. Headache

This symptom was recorded on 159 occasions (89 females; 70 males). It was rare under the age of 5 years. The highest rates occurred in both males and females between the ages of 5 and 24 years. Higher rates were recorded by patients in social classes III, IV, and V than in social classes I and II. The diagnoses recorded were:

Diagnosis	Number of consultations
Psychiatric disorders	31
Acute sinusitis	26
Migraine	19
Tonsillitis	12
Common cold	6
Influenza	3
Benign hypertension	3
Refractive errors	2
Others	57
Total	159

10. Joint pains

This symptom was recorded on 141 occasions (75 females; 66 males). The highest rates were recorded in females over the age of 45 years. Between the ages of 5 and 44 years, higher rates were recorded in males than in females. This symptom was recorded more frequently in social classes III, IV, and V than in social classes I and II. The diagnoses recorded were:

Diagnosis	Number of consultations
Sprains and strains	25
Osteoarthritis	25
Arthritis (unspecified)	17
Contusions and superficial abrasions	14
Fibrositis and muscular rheumatism	6
Rheumatoid arthritis	5
Synovitis	5
Psychiatric disorders	3
Gout	3
Others	38
Total	141

11. Disturbance of gastric function

This symptom was recorded on 141 occasions (80 females; 61 males). The highest rates occurred in patients under the age of 5 years in which the symptom was twice as common as in any other age group. This symptom became less common with increasing age. The highest rate of presentation of this symptom occurred in patients in social classes I and II. The diagnoses recorded were:

Diagnosis	Number of consultations
Other diseases of the stomach and duodenum	44
Symptomatic diagnosis (vomiting)	25
Other diseases of the intestine and peritoneum	10

Disorders of gastric function	9
Tonsillitis	8
Common cold	6
Psychiatric disorders	6
Pregnancy	3
Others	30
Total	141

12. Disturbance of balance

This system was recorded at 74 consultations (52 females; 22 males) thus showing a marked female preponderance. The highest rates were recorded in females over the age of 65 years and the rate for females was higher than that of males in all age groups. The diagnoses recorded were:

Diagnosis	Number of consultations
Symptomatic diagnosis (vertigo)	17
Psychiatric disorder	16
Vascular lesion of the CNS	5
Benign hypertension	4
Ménière's disease	2
Motion sickness	2
Wax in the ears	2
Others	26
Total	74

13. Changes in energy, and tiredness

This symptom was recorded on 58 occasions (43 females; 15 males); again there was a marked female preponderance. The highest rates were recorded in females between the ages of 15 and 64 years. The diagnoses recorded were:

Diagnosis	Number of consultations
Psychiatric disorder	30
Hypochromic anaemia	4
Common cold	3
Influenza	3
Pregnancy	2
Others	16
Total	58

14. Disturbance of breathing

This symptom was recorded at 61 consultations (29 females; 32 males). The highest rates were recorded in males aged 15–24 years and in both males and females over the age of 65 years. The diagnoses recorded were:

Diagnosis	Number of consultations
Acute bronchitis	16
Common cold	13
Chronic bronchitis	7
Psychiatric disorders	5
Asthma	3
Hypochromic anaemia	2
Benign hypertension	2
Others	13
Total	61

5

History taking in general practice

In Chapter 4 the various diagnostic models used in medicine have been explained. All of these depend on the collection and interpretation of information provided by patients.

There is increasing emphasis on the acquisition of communication skills in medical schools throughout the world, and in postgraduate education. The drive for this new initiative has often come from departments of general practice. Asking why this should be so leads to answers that illustrate important characteristics of general practice. The man who is referred to a specialist complaining of, for example, epigastric pain that is relieved by food and wakens him in the early hours of the morning, might need investigating but not sophisticated communication skills; likewise, the patient referred to the specialist with a lump in the groin, which has a positive cough impulse, or the patient with typical cardiac pain on exercise that is now occurring at rest. Good communication skills are much more necessary when faced with a patient with unexplained fatigue, a band-like headache interfering with work and social activities, or recurrent diarrhoea following a family crisis.

The accessibility of general practitioners means that they are concerned with: evaluating the early signs of illness; separating the normal from the abnormal; exploring why a patient has consulted at a particular point in time in terms of the physical, social, and psychological stresses to which that patient is exposed; and with all those factors that influence patients in seeking medical care that were described in Chapter 3.

COMMUNICATION SKILLS

It is at this stage in the provision of medical care that skills in communication are most important. About one half of consultations in general practice are concerned with new problems. The way in which the problem is presented depends on the patient's interpretation of the symptoms of illness that they have experienced. This is influenced by their previous experience of illness, discussions with family and neighbours, health beliefs, and a wide variety of other factors. The doctor's task is to identify what patients have experienced and why this has led them to consult at a particular point in time. The probabilty of identifying a patient's main problem and anxiety is related to the dialogue that takes place between patient and doctor in the consultation.

In general practice the doctor usually enters a consultation with the considerable advantage that this forms part of an ongoing relationship. The doctor might have known the patient for a number of years, know the social background, have made some assessment of the patient's personality and their threshold for consulting, and might have visited the patient's home. Equally the patient knows the doctor, and this might influence the way in which problems are presented. A long and trusting relationship may lead to the presentation of problems in a more open way than is possible when no pre-existing relationship exists.

Communication is concerned with more than just the dialogue that takes place in the consultation. A great deal of information can be gleaned from the way in which the patient enters the consulting room. The patient might enter with a slow, painful, unsteady, or unusual gait. Their expression might display pleasure, anxiety, or long suffering. When invited to sit down they might lower themselves painfully into the seat or express a preference for standing, a common physical sign of a prolapsed or thrombosed pile, perineal abscess, or coccydynia. The patient might sit staring at the floor to avoid eye contact, with arms crossed or fingering the nose or face, all of which reflect insecurity. Alternatively, they might adopt an open position with good eye contact and smiles. Some patients might be effusive, apologizing for taking up the doctor's time, but talking incessantly; others might be monosyllabic thus presenting serious problems with opening up any sort of dialogue. The former might be attention seeking and the latter depressed. The way in which the patient moves might also convey important messages to the doctor. The patient with severe abdominal or pleuritic pain moves with great economy of effort, showing clear evidence of pain on movement; the patient with serious shortness of breath reduces verbal communication to short sentences and monosyllables; the pyrexial adult or child is subdued, moves slowly, and often responds to questions in a monotone. In contrast, attention seeking patients explain their symptoms with enthusiasm and melodramatic gestures.

Skills in communication are therefore concerned not only with dialogue between patient and doctor but also with simple observations of the patient, which frequently communicate most important messages.

VERBAL COMMUNICATION

Skills in verbal communication are particularly concerned with the ability of doctors to encourage patients to express their problems and feelings in their own words. It has been said that questions produce answers, but the relevance of these answers is often questionable. In communicating with patients the objectives should be firstly, to encourage patients to describe what they have noticed wrong, secondly, to find out how this affects them, and thirdly, to find out what anxieties have been provoked. Questions should be open-ended, for example 'Tell me about it'; 'What do you feel is the problem?'; 'How do you feel about it?'; 'How do you think I can help?'; 'Tell me about your marriage / bowels / sleep pattern / sexual relationships'. At the end of the consultation some closed questions might be needed, but these should always be offered to the patient as alternatives such as, 'Is your appetite better or worse than it was 2 months ago?'; 'Are you more or less breathless climbing the stairs to your flat than you were this time last year?'.

Sometimes patients experience difficulty in expressing their problems or responding to the doctor's open-ended questions. A period of silence might ensue, which the doctor is sorely tempted to end by another question. Silence, however, can be of immense value in identifying patient's problems and should always be respected. It will often lead to new and important information. In contrast, particularly when interviewed by medical students, the patient might indulge in a monologue, which can cause some difficulty because the student does not know how to intervene. To bring this under control, it is often helpful for the doctor or student to interject and say 'Let me try to summarize your problem'.

Some patients experience great difficulty in describing their symptoms and anxieties. Doctors must then use their skills to encourage communication and here body language is important. The doctors' position is relevant—they should sit back, appear relaxed with their arms open, inviting communication. The patient's description of the symptoms or feelings must draw a response in terms of 'umms' or 'ahas' and at times it might be helpful to repeat the last few words of the patient's statement, such as:

Patient: 'My husband just doesn't understand'

Doctor: 'Your husband doesn't understand'

Patient: 'My daughter wants to lead her own life'

Doctor: 'Your daughter wants to lead her own life'

These various techniques are known as facilitation and are important skills to acquire in promoting good doctor–patient communications. These communications are not simply concerned with words or with the 'umms' and 'ahas' but also with conveying empathy to the patient. It is important to let patients know that doctors really care about their problems and that they are prepared to be non-judgemental.

Many academic departments of general practice train undergraduates in these skills by arranging for them to interview real patients and to indulge in role play exercises. Not uncommonly these 'consultations' are tape or video recorded so that students can retrospectively study their own consultation techniques.

It is sometimes claimed, and there is some research experience to support this, that in 90 per cent of cases doctors make their diagnosis on the basis of the medical history alone, and in only 10 per cent do the results of physical examination or investigation contribute to the diagnostic process. This will, however, obviously vary with the skill of the doctor in eliciting a good history.

No doctor, in the course of the short consultation characteristic of general practice in the United Kingdom, can be expected to elicit all the information needed to make management decisions. This is where another characteristic of general practice, continuity of care, is so important. Information about patients, their families, and social background that has been accumulated over months or years, can be used in the context of new information and new episodes of illness presented.

Good history taking or communication facilitates the acquisition of new information. In general practice, this can be set against a background of information, which might be held in the doctor's memory, or be made overt in good medical records. In a group practice when different doctors might be consulted in an emergency, good records are of great importance.

It is helpful to develop a record system that displays the relationships within a family. Ideally this should be illustrated graphically so that doctors may quickly obtain the information they require. Such a system has been described by Cormack (1975) and is illustrated in Fig. 5.1. Pictorial relationships of members of the family are prepared by a clerical worker from a simple questionnaire completed by all newly registering families. It is added to when the practice receives the patient's previous records from the Family Health Services Authority and is regularly updated. A photocopy can be kept in the records of each member of the family. In some practices it is customary to file the records of all members of a family together and this again provides the doctor with an opportunity to relate illness in one family member to the family as a whole.

Histories taken by general practitioners are particularly important because they are the first doctors to listen to patients' stories. By the time patients have recited their histories to their own doctors, have had them accepted, and have been referred to a hospital, these histories are likely to be well organized in patients' minds. This makes subsequent history taking easier, but such histories might not be so closely related to what patients are really experiencing. At the first consultation doctors might ask leading questions or give complaints provisional diagnoses, and doubtless patients will then discuss this further with their family and friends. Diagnostically, the first history that the general practitioner takes is therefore often the most valuable.

The skill of seeing a symptom as a variation in a patient's life rather than something new, can only be developed by the doctor who is privileged to watch the lives for whom he is responsible as they develop under the pressures of the environment and disease. It is an art acquired gradually and almost sub-consciously. Doctors fit the troubles of their patients into their mental picture of their patients lives. Something might then suddenly occur that will not harmonize with the background, like a discord in the middle of a

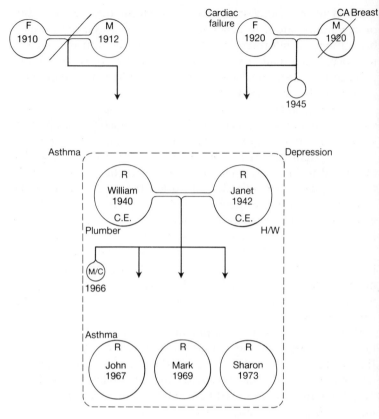

Fig. 5.1. Record card summarizing the relationships within a family (From Cormack, J. J. C., (1975). Family portraits. *Journal of the Royal College of Practitioners*, **25**, 520.)

symphony, and they become alert and realize that something is wrong. This is the scenario into which medical students are introduced in their clerkships in general practice.

This ability to pick out the significant from much that is insignificant can be observed at any time in the surgery work of a good family doctor. It is not something that can be taught easily. Some examples might clarify this.

Case 17. Miss F. complained to the doctor that she had a sore throat and had felt sick on and off for about a week. Examination showed only slight redness of the pharynx. She was a girl of 20 whom the doctor knew well, having been to the home on many occasions. She rarely consulted him for minor ailments and though she did not look ill on this occasion, her behaviour was peculiarly subdued. Instead of ending the interview with advice on the use of aspirin, the doctor said, 'Come on Pat, what's worrying you?' It transpired that she had missed two periods. Did the doctor think this was due to changing her job?

Case 18. Mrs P. came to the doctor complaining of having felt tired and depressed for 2 months. He had delivered her of two children and knew her to be a well balanced woman with a happy home. A full history and examination showed no abnormality, but these symptoms did not fit in with the doctor's mental picture of Mrs P's life. Further investigation was carried out, which showed that she had sarcoidosis.

Case 19. Mrs J. also complained of tiredness. She was married with four young children and her husband was a salesman who was often away from home. She had been a teacher before her marriage and did not take kindly to being chained to the kitchen sink. For some years she had needed intermittent medical support and her new complaint fitted into the doctor's previous experience of his patient. She was allowed to talk about her troubles.

In addition to the facility that doctors develop for detecting anomalous situations, knowledge about patients also helps doctors to come to the subject of the consultation more quickly. The fact that they and their patients are acquainted reduces the frequency with which consultations are confused by embarrassment or fear. Many patients go to their doctor if they want time off work. It might seem incongruous that Mr D., a strong independent man, should come to his doctor with a cold. If, however, it is known that Mr D. works in the open air as a railway labourer, that there is snow on the ground, and he needs time off work, it becomes more understandable. If, in addition, Mr D. knows that he can say this to his doctor and get what he wants without reciting a stream of symptoms to prove his point, it will save a lot of time.

Despite these advantages however, general practitioners often experience difficulty in selecting those patients with whom they should devote time and those with whom they can deal more expeditiously. The answer to the question 'Why has this patient come to see me at this point in time?' will be self-evident in many consultations for acute illness. There will, however, always be situations when some anomaly arouses the doctor's suspicions. For this reason, doctors should, even in the most trivial of cases, give patients the opportunity to say more if they wish to do so. A remark such as 'Were you perfectly well before this trouble started?', or 'Have you any other problems?', might be all that is necessary to open the flood gates to a stream of pent-up anxiety.

Students attached to general practitioners will have no past knowledge of the patients to work on and will therefore often be confused by the clinical interviews they observe. A few students unfortunately give up at this stage. Because the doctor does not take the sort of history and perform the full examination that they have learned to respect as 'proper medicine', they cease to understand medicine at all. They fail to realize that general practice demands special skills and that the hospital diagnostic model is not always applicable. In general practice it is necessary to know everybody so that the person who is ill can be picked out like a weed in a bunch of flowers. Once you become familiar with the flowers, it is easier to see which one is different. The first week or two in general practice is often confusing.

It might be helpful to try to summarize the way in which general practitioners approach their surgery consultations, but the following observations will be of value only if it is appreciated, as will become apparent subsequently, that there are many exceptions.

1. In patients with acute illnesses and acute trauma a very short history will usually suffice unless there is some obvious incongruity, for example, excessive complaining about minor trauma; pyrexia in the absence of any other symptoms.

2. Patients newly joining the practice need a history that is designed to make some estimate of them as people and to identify their medical history and social situation.

3. Patients who rarely consult the doctor should, if possible, be dealt with at one consultation. The more vague the presenting symptoms, the more exhaustive must be the history. These patients cannot be depended on to come back if symptomatic treatment is unsuccessful.

4. Complaints of patients known to have serious underlying disease are considered against this background. Most of these patients are, however, used to attending regularly and can be depended on to return at a later date if the doctor is busy.

5. Mothers with young families can usually be treated expeditiously and will return readily for review. A mother on her

own might, however, belittle her symptoms. If the doctor is pressed for time, arranging a visit at home to give the patient more time will often provide valuable information, and will help to establish a relationship with the children.

6. With children under the age of 6 years, time given to history taking from the mother allows the child to become accustomed to the doctor and makes subsequent examination easier.

7. Every doctor is faced with a few patients who go from one doctor to another. They usually give the impression that they have had a poor deal in the past but that the new doctor is different and more up-to-date etc. They are usually attention seeking but will need a full evaluation before limits are set to their demands.

8. The chronic 'high users' are often dealt with expeditiously, but an opportunity should be made at some time to give them full consideration, preferably after consultation with a partner, in an attempt to elucidate why they behave in this way.

The infinite variety of disease, both in type and severity, that is presented to the family doctor, demands an elasticity of mind and method that is not required elsewhere in medicine. Though it is impossible to develop a stereotyped approach to even the commonest problems, it is necessary to develop a technique for dealing with certain symptoms. When dealing with twenty or thirty patients complaining of backache who have no serious underlying pathology, it is easy to slip into an imperfect form of history-taking. The characteristics, time relationships, etc. of pain that are learned as a student can quickly be forgotten when they have proved excessively detailed on many occasions. Yet general practitioners who depend so largely on history-taking, must make the greatest possible use of the patients' descriptions of their diseases. The factor that constantly controls the extent to which the doctor falls short of the ideal, is time. In the winter there might be insufficient time in the day to give proper attention to all the problems encountered, but even in the slack periods, time will often be short at that moment when a new problem is presented. This is usually in the surgery when it is difficult to give a prolonged consultation while others are waiting. There are various ways of dealing with this situation, but in general practice when the demands on the doctor's time are so unpredictable and under the influence of such things as epidemics and weather conditions, there is no simple answer.

The arrangement of an appointment system helps to solve the problem, but it requires additional secretarial assistance and, unless 10 minutes can be assigned to every new patient, there will be many occasions when it will not be possible to achieve a satisfactory result in the time available. I have shown that more problems are identified when more time is available (Morrell *et al.* 1986). Doctors both with and without appointment systems will therefore be faced with some patients who have to be asked to return at a later date for more thorough consideration of their problems. This has the disadvantage that the doctor cannot 'strike while the iron is hot'. On the other hand, it is often helpful to doctors because it gives them time to prepare for particular problems.

Some doctors like to deal with every problem as completely as possible when it is presented, but they must steel themselves to the patients who are sitting in the waiting-room and be prepared to have surgeries that go on for a long time. Others like to elicit their histories piecemeal, if necessary at several consultations. This has the doubtful advantage that those patients with less serious pathology will probably recover completely with symptomatic treatment without the necessity for a full history, but it lacks continuity and might give the patient the impression that the doctor's approach is rather casual.

Appointment systems are used by most doctors and patients in the United Kingdom. When properly organized they can cope with fluctuations in demand without creating waiting lists, and they can also allow doctors the freedom to book patients for blocks of time if they feel that this is desirable. They certainly reduce the time patients wait to see their doctor. History taking in the patient's home rarely presents the problems that arise in a consultation at the doctor's surgery. Most new calls to the home are concerned with acute illness or acute episodes in chronic illness. Although there might be unnecessary house calls, the problems presented are usually clear cut and doctors are more easily able to assess what is required of them and respond appropriately. In addition, the doctor is less pressed in the patient's home than in the surgery, and a temporary hold-up on his round can be redressed by hurrying through some of the less serious subsequent visits. Nevertheless, many of the questions that will now be considered concerning history-taking are applicable to consultations made in the home as well as to those made in the doctor's surgery.

WHAT IS THE PATIENT'S PROBLEM?

The most important fact to establish is what is it that the patient is experiencing? The ease with which this is achieved is not necessarily related to the intelligence of the patient. The symptom presented is in the form of a tentative offer to the doctor. It has usually been the subject of considerable thought and is framed in such a way that it interests and possibly impresses the doctor, but at the same time, preserves the dignity of the patient. Many patients do not feel comfortable with simple undecorated symptoms. A chill in the stomach, bladder, or bowel is preferred to vomiting, pain on passing water, or diarrhoea. A touch of rheumatism is considered more respectable than a stiff or painful joint, and a 'cold' might mean anything from a nasal discharge to a vaginal one and involve any of the organs that lie between. This desire to present a diagnosis can be confusing and occasionally dangerous as the following case histories demonstrate.

Case 20. Mrs M. requested a call at 10.00pm on a Saturday. She was aged 50 and complaining of hot flushes. The doctor was a little irritated by such a complaint at that time and was loath to leave his fireside. The neighbour, however, insisted that he should come and reluctantly he agreed. The patient, who had not previously been seen by the doctor, was found to be suffering from pneumonia. She was indeed suffering from hot flushes due to a life threatening infection.

Case 21. Mr L., aged 19, was complaining of severe abdominal pain. 'Would the doctor come at once?' He called about thirty minutes later, having interrupted his surgery, to find the patient sitting comfortably by the fire. The history disclosed that the cascara had now produced the desired result with great relief all round.

Case 22. Mrs J. attended the surgery complaining of a cold in the chest. The history disclosed that her main symptom was pain in the chest, but she said that this was a not severe pain and she would not have come if her husband had not insisted. With further questioning it transpired that the pain was not really worrying her at all, but she had noticed a lump in her breast. Examination showed a carcinoma of the breast.

These examples could be multiplied almost indefinitely, but they emphasize the importance of knowing exactly what the patient means. Not only is this necessary for accurate diagnoses to be made but is essential if valuable time is to be saved. Every doctor with experience in general practice will remember the embarrassing occasions when he has not taken enough trouble to elicit the presenting symptoms.

Case 23. Mr R. attended evening surgery complaining of a touch of indigestion. 'Perhaps you could give me a bottle just to settle it'. The bottle was prescribed with a proviso that he should return in a week if he was not better. A week later he was rather worse. Further enquiry disclosed that Mr R's indigestion was in fact a gripping, retrosternal sensation 'and now that you come to mention it, doctor, it is worse when I hurry'.

Certain symptoms are notorious in this respect. Indigestion, a touch of rheumatism, a cold or chill anywhere, and the feeling of being run down, are perhaps some of the most dangerous. In probably 80 per cent of cases the trouble will not be serious, but that is why general practice is so difficult and so interesting.

Having ascertained what has brought the patient to consult his doctor, half the battle is over. If the patient and the real reason for consultation are known, it is usually possible to immediately decide the seriousness with which the particular problem should be tackled. This is the secret of successful history-taking in general practice; a high degree of selection occurs at an early stage in each consultation.

The following examples are of three patients, seen in one day, complaining of headache.

Case 24. Mr H., aged 30, complained of a right frontal headache of 3 days duration. He was known to the doctor and rarely visited the surgery. Some fairly direct questioning elicited that the headache was intermittent, worse on bending and coughing, and was associated with a nasal discharge and tenderness over both antra. The interview was completed inside 5 minutes.

Case 25. Mrs D., aged 34, said 'I feel dreadful doctor'. Questioning disclosed that, apart from her usual exhaustion, she had had a terrible headache for 5 days, from which she had had no respite. Mrs D., in spite of her terrible sufferings, remained in excellent physical condition. Her family life was known to the doctor to be miserable and not amenable to treatment. History-taking was kept at a superficial level and Mrs D left, armed with an analgesic, within 5 minutes.

Case 26. Mr J., aged 54, complained of a frontal headache that troubled him in the evenings. The doctor had never met him before although he had seen his wife and daughter. His symptoms had been present for 3 weeks. Mr J. was given a 20 minute appointment for a few days later and left within 3 minutes. At the subsequent interview a full history and examination were completed.

Analysing the doctor's thoughts in dealing with the above patients will throw some light on the approach to history-taking in general practice. When the first patient entered the consulting-room, the doctor would know that this was a man who rarely consulted and therefore must be taken seriously. His illness is acute and his symptoms clear cut, and the doctor would think 'I can solve this problem here and now and give this patient immediate relief'. The second patient would be received with a heavy heart. The doctor will have tried unsuccessfully to cure her in the past so that they now have an unspoken agreement between themselves. She presents the symptoms, the doctor provides a remedy, and both remain tolerably happy. With the third patient the doctor would think 'I don't know this man and I haven't a hope of sorting him out in the time available. His symptoms have been present for 3 weeks and so it will pay in the long run to give him more time when it is convenient'.

Case 24 is the easiest to deal with but there are certain difficulties, even with this type of case. Many of the problems seen by the family doctor are minor so that, even with a clear cut presenting symptom, it is easy to forget the importance of the history. It is much quicker to say to the patient with pain in the chest 'Take your shirt off' than to ask a few questions about the pain. Yet examination is usually much less rewarding. For all the common symptoms the doctor should have a mental list of the factors that must be elicited. The patient should be allowed to tell his own story and the doctor then ask such questions as are necessary to complete the picture.

The type of case illustrated by case 25 will be considered later in this chapter. Case 26 has many similarities to the patient seen in hospital. He is a stranger to the family doctor who therefore cannot use his or her most valuable tool, knowledge of the patient, in assessing the new symptom. If busy, the doctor might be tempted to temporize with a cursory examination, but hours will be saved in the long run by getting to know the patient. The knowledge thus gained, if not of value in solving the current problem, will undoubtedly be drawn on at subsequent consultations.

DIFFIDENCE IN CONSULTING THE DOCTOR

Most patients experience some diffidence or shyness in approaching the doctor and there are at least three factors that play a part in this. Probably the most important is the difficulty that the layman has in finding words to convey to the doctor what he or she is experiencing. A lady who suffers a burning retrosternal pain that awakens her at night and causes acute discomfort and heartburn when weeding the garden, might become confused when she tries to put this into words that she understands. It might be described as indigestion, a feeling that she is going to choke, sickness, or a cold in the chest. If the doctor accepts the presenting symptoms without question then the wrong conclusion might be reached.

The second difficulty is caused by the fact that certain functions of the body, mainly those concerned with excretion and reproduction, are shrouded in modesty, which, not unbecoming in the drawing-room, can be a source of great confusion in the consulting room.

Pride plays a big part in deciding which symptoms the patient will present to the doctor. Certain symptoms are considered rather unworthy and will often only be elicited by questioning. The following examples illustrate some of these problems.

Case 27. Mrs L., aged 24, complained of pain when passing urine. Further questioning elicited that her real complaint was a vaginal discharge. Examination did not show an excessive discharge, but did show that the patient was a virgin. She had been married for 3 months and discussion disclosed that she had failed to consummate her marriage. This, she admitted, was the real reason for the consultation; the presenting symptoms being designed to direct her doctor to a symptom that she simply could not bring herself to discuss.

Case 28. Mr J., aged 54, came to the doctor complaining of a cough. Examination showed no abnormality and he was treated symptomatically. At the next consultation his cough was no better and he mentioned that he was also constipated. The following day Mrs J. also consulted the doctor with a cough, but mentioned that her husband had been passing blood per rectum. At the third attempt the doctor was successful in eliciting the real reason for the consultation. Further investigation disclosed a rectal carcinoma.

Case 29. Mr R., a rather arrogant and successful business man, came to the doctor for a tonic. He hadn't felt really fit since having 'flu' 2 months before. To the doctor's surprise, after answering a few questions mono-syllabically, which suggested that they should never have been asked, Mr R. began to cry. For years he had considered mental illness as a sign of weakness and was unable to face up to the fact that he was mentally ill.

The methods adopted by patients to overcome their shyness are often a source of surprise to the doctor. Some consider all illness a sign of weakness and, as in case 29, they are quite likely to approach the doctor in an arrogant and demanding manner, compensating for their insecurity by a show of strength. Doctors nearly always find this alarming and they might react in a similar manner as they in turn become insecure, imagining that patients regard them as weak and ready to be trampled on. This can cause unfortunate situations to arise and therefore doctors must try to react by asking 'Why do these people behave in such an extraordinary way?' rather than by reacting aggressively themselves.

In addition to shyness, modesty, and pride, another potent source of confusion is fear. This most commonly is a fear of the diagnosis, but might occasionally be fear of the doctor.

Case 30. Mrs K. complained of a most curious sensation of unreality that she had experienced in short attacks for about 6 months. On one occasion she had lost consciousness. She had not come to consult the doctor earlier because she was afraid he would laugh at her and think she was fussing. Further questioning suggested that these were epileptic manifestations and she was investigated for a cerebral tumour.

A combination of shyness and fear of the doctor seemed to be the cause of this late consultation, and it was a reflection on the doctor that she could not confide more easily. Patients vary greatly in this respect and though some often consult the doctor unnecessarily, it is always rather embarrassing for the doctor to see a seriously ill patient after an excessive delay because 'We know you are so busy doctor'. One wonders if the busy doctor is not perhaps overplayed at times.

Fear of the diagnosis is, however, a much more common cause of difficulty in history-taking. Cancer is the most feared disease, but occasionally high blood pressure, stroke, or a less common disease is the cause. There can be no doubt that many curable neoplasms are left until too late because of fear. In some cases patients might simply not report to doctors; in others they try to mislead them, hoping in some obscure way, that they will find some other explanation for their symptoms.

Case 31. Mrs K., aged 70, asked the doctor to visit because she had a sore on her chest that needed dressing. Examination disclosed a fungating carcinoma that had been present for about 5 years, but was now so infected that she was compelled to seek advice.

Case 32. Mrs P. complained that she felt run down and needed a tonic. She was a strong woman who, despite having a large family that was now nearly off her hands, rarely bothered the doctor. This fortunately aroused his suspicions and questioning elicited two episodes of intermenstrual bleeding. Examination disclosed an early carcinoma of the cervix, which fortunately responded well to radiotherapy and Mrs P. is, after 5 years, apparently cured.

Case 33. Mr H. was a chronic bronchitic, aged 50. He complained of shortness of breath that was not a new symptom. This made the doctor wonder why he had bothered to mention it. Further questioning disclosed little else until, just as he was leaving, he mentioned that he had coughed up some blood the day before. He was terrified of cancer, but fortunately further investigation was negative.

Fear is occasionally instrumental in making a patient complain of symptoms that will, if this fear is removed, disappear entirely. Raised blood pressure is perhaps the commonest of these, particularly in middle-aged women.

Case 34. Mrs T., aged 52, complained of headaches and attacks of giddiness. It transpired that her father had had high blood pressure and had died from a stroke, and that her friend had just been told that she suffered from this condition. When Mrs T. was reassured that her blood pressure was normal, she was relieved of her symptoms, which did not recur.

Most serious and even rare diseases produce common symptoms, such as, abdominal pain, pains in the chest, or cough. While well-balanced patients appreciate this and do not immediately fear the worst, some more imaginative individuals always see their symptoms as the same as 'so and so' who was dead 3 months later. Fear might either drive them to the doctor with every trivial complaint or keep them away for fear of the diagnosis.

Case 35. Stella B., aged 5, had tonsillitis. The doctor called and having looked at the child's throat, was astonished to see the mother standing, pale and crying, at the foot of the bed. 'Is it leukaemia doctor?' she managed to blurt out. When reassured that it was not, she was overcome with relief and gratitude—she'd read it in the papers only the other day etc.

Sometimes it is difficult for doctors to know whether it is shyness, fear, or sheer stupidity that is obstructing their history-taking. Many doctors regard the first two sympathetically, but stupidity is something for which the patient is to blame. In point of fact, however, it is the most excusable. In practice, stupidity as it appears in the mentally subnormal, is much less of a problem than the type that is a product of education that endows the individual with limited knowledge. A patient might say outright, or infer, 'I don't want to tell you your job doctor, but...' or 'Well that is funny because my friend had precisely these symptoms and his man in Harley Street said it was so and so'. Such patients make their symptom fit their diagnosis and then present doctors with an edited version. This militates against an accurate diagnosis in two ways. Firstly, doctors might become angry, and secondly, it makes it difficult to find out exactly what these patients are experiencing.

Case 36. Mrs D. consulted the doctor because she said that she had a cancer of the bowel. She had had diarrhoea for 1 week, accompanied by 'excruciating' abdominal pains. 'Exactly like my mother who died of cancer'. The diarrhoea did not respond to simple treatment and the stools were cultured without finding pathogens. After a further week of treatment, however, the symptoms abated. During this time Mr D. confided that his wife was neurotic and he was sick and tired of her bowels. One week later Mr D. announced that he had a slipped disc. There were no signs to confirm this diagnosis but for 2 weeks he lay flat on his back complaining of pain. The doctor was so emotionally involved with the family by now that any attempt to sort out their problems was doomed to failure. He capitulated, sent Mr D. into hospital and within 2 days he was symptom-free. He was subsequently discharged with the diagnosis of slipped disc, which he proudly announced to his doctor. The doctor was still convinced that Mr D.'s illness was hysterical and the encounter hardly improved the doctor–patient relationship.

This case illustrates many problems but is included here to show that if the doctor had not reacted adversely to Mrs D.'s original high-handed diagnostic approach but had tried to find out what was bothering her from the start, a lot of trouble might have been saved.

Patients who like to present doctors with diagnoses are particularly irritating. Doctors might find it hard to accept a diagnosis if it is at variance with the presenting symptoms and signs. They might be tempted to refute it, which might bring the retort that numerous

X-rays and specialists have been consulted in the past to verify the diagnosis and the usually unspoken query 'Who are you to question such eminent authorities?' It is wise in such cases to remember that some people find it necessary to go through life labelled as a martyr to sinusitis or colitis. It is not, of course, a diagnosis in the scientific sense, but it is serving a useful purpose and it will often do harm to both patient and doctor if it is destroyed.

It follows that history-taking must not only determine what the patient is experiencing but also what sort of person is experiencing these symptoms. This knowledge might already be available to the doctor or be obtainable from medical records. Alternatively, a few well-directed questions will often given some indications. School record will give an idea of intelligence; work record might suggest instability; the inside of a patient's house might provide evidence of an obsessional, slovenly, or overworked housewife; patients' pastimes will help to assess whether they are essentially extroverted or introverted; patients' accounts of their medical histories and experiences with doctors will often disclose those who have hysterical personalities or those who are prone to bouts of depression.

The next chapter is concerned with the examination of patients, but it is important to stress that an overall assessment of personalities is made not only from what the patients say but also from their general behaviour. The monosyllabic response and neglected dress of the depressed patient; the defensive posture, with arms and legs crossed, of the insecure patient who avoids eye-to-eye contact; the flirtatious of effusive approach of the hysteric; or the restlessness of the anxious patient. All these observations and many more tell general practitioners about the sorts of people who are consulting them.

An attempt should always be made to establish a tentative diagnosis of a patient's personality, which can then be modified in the light of subsequent experience. It might be totally irrelevant to the current problem, but it is surprising how commonly diagnosis and treatment are influenced by the type of person concerned. Occasionally a more thorough psychiatric assessment might be indicated.

HISTORY-TAKING IN CHILDREN

With adults, history-taking concerns the actions and reactions of only two people, the doctor and the patient. With children, however, who account for much of the workload of family doctors', a third person becomes involved. The technique in dealing with children varies with the age of the patient. Doctors should encourage children to form independent relationships with them as early as possible, because children who are familiar with their doctors and able to answer simple questions, can provide more accurate accounts of what they are experiencing than most adults, whose experiences are often coloured by imagination and pre-conceived ideas. Normal, co-operative, friendly children can make useful contributions to their histories from the age of about 5 years.

Before this age, history-taking must be done largely through an intermediary, usually the mother. When dealing with children, it is always worth spending several minutes on history-taking, however busy the surgery or trivial the complaint. This gives the child time to get used to the surroundings, to inspect the doctor, and to gain confidence by seeing an easy relationship between mother and doctor. During this time, it is often best to ignore the child. This will save time and trouble in subsequent encounters, the only exceptions being babies up to 6 months old or children who are so familiar with the doctor that such a preparation is unnecessary.

The object of the history is the same as with adults, to determine what the patient is experiencing and why this particular consultation has occurred at this particular time. Though the parent can usually give an answer to the second part of this question, the first part depends on the mother's account of the abnormalities that she has noticed or that have been conveyed to her by the child. Her value as an interpreter is a reflection on her ability as a mother, rather than a product of education or the result of a prolonged study of baby books or womens' magazines. As a rule, more difficulty is experienced by mothers with their first baby and by mothers who come from small families. In these days, a term such as 'instinct' is hardly acceptable, but most doctors appreciate that good mothers know instinctively when their babies are ill, and good family doctors know by experience who are the good mothers in their practices. Some mothers never seem to get closer to their children than an arm's length and might be oblivious to the severity of their child's illness on one occasion, yet on another make an enormous fuss over some trifling abnormality.

There are certain characteristics of normal babies that are notoriously liable to misinterpretation. When babies cry they often draw their legs up. Adults, however, draw up their legs in response to abdominal pain and mothers therefore often say that 'The baby has the most terrible colic, doctor'. When normal babies suck teats with a small hole they quickly tire, swallow air, and become annoyed, particularly when, having brought up wind, they find their stomachs empty. Mothers then say that they won't take their feeds and that they are screaming with tummy pains. Teething infants often experience pain in the ear and might therefore rub their ears. Mothers might take such infants to the doctor saying that they have earache. The baby might have a sore mouth and be presented with loss of appetite, sore throat, or screaming attacks.

Toddlers who discover how solicitous their mothers become if they refuse to eat will be brought to the doctor for a tonic to improve their appetite. 'My little boy wakes up screaming with pain, doctor' might indicate either that he has discovered that by doing so he can be taken into his mother's bed, or that his anus is itching because he has got threadworms.

These examples show how fallible symptoms are in children when interpreted by a third person, and it is very important for the doctor to know precisely what the mother has noticed. Having achieved this, the interpretation of symptoms in children under the age of 5 is still difficult. For example, a simple infection such as tonsillitis might present under the guise of loss of appetite, abdominal pain, vomiting, or simple pyrexia. In the older age groups, a child, if given the opportunity, will often be able to point to the seat of the trouble more precisely, although limitation of vocabulary may lead to confusion. Thus 'pain in the tummy' may indicate pain anywhere from the neck to the pelvis. It is important to try to encourage the child from an early age to become an active party in eliciting the history and to educate the parents to allow the child the degree of independence that this requires. It is not, of course, opportune to initiate such training during an illness and therefore the doctor should be prepared to invest time to do this during consultations of minor importance when the child is in a co-operative frame of mind.

The significance of symptoms reported by a parent must always be assessed in the context of the whole family. When a mother has been neglectful to a child she might make light of serious ill health in an attempt to justify her own neglect. On the other hand, the mother who likes to relinquish responsibility for every trivial upset in her children will frequently exaggerate the symptoms and turn even minor illness into an acute emergency.

Occasionally the child is made the presenting symptom by a parent who wishes to consult the doctor about a problem that she does not feel can be presented alone. The remark, 'While I am here, doctor' often means 'Why I am here'.

Case 37. Mrs V. brought her baby son to the doctor because she thought that his eczema was becoming worse. His skin, however, appeared unchanged and enquiries about life in general disclosed that Mrs V. would like 'something for her nerves'. It transpired that Mr V. had left home the previous week with an unmarried girl from the next village.

The patient who consults a doctor in hospital is regarded as an individual and a diagnosis is usually reached without going deeply into the patient's environment. The general practitioner must, however, regard every patient as a member of his community and see each one as a member of a family of which he has at least made some assessment. This is an enormous advantage in evaluating symptoms in adults and essential in children. Only rarely can an illness be regarded as a clear-cut entity with a beginning and an end. More often it is a deviation from normal produced by a number of factors acting over a period of time and with implications that reach outside the individual concerned. Family doctors are ideally placed to appreciate all dimensions of illness and they should train themselves to think in this way at each stage in the diagnostic process.

REFERENCES

Cormack, J. J. C. (1975). Family portraits. *Journal of the Royal College of General Practitioners*, **25**, 520.

Morrell, D., Evans, M., Morris, R., and Roland, M. (1986). The 'Five minute consultation': the effect of time constraint on clinical content and patient satisfaction. *British Medical Journal*, **292**, 870–3.

6

Examination of the patient in general practice

All medical students are taught how to carry out a full physical examination of a patient. All the main systems of the body are explored and they learn how to become familiar with the normal to enable them to identify the abnormal. This usually takes place in hospital wards where patients are available in bed and it is easy to carry out this examination and where many of the patients have signs of clinical abnormalities. This is a most important part in the training of medical students and the sooner students acquire these basic skills the more they will be able to perfect them in their subsequent training. As students work through the out-patient departments they will observe that the performing of the comprehensive clinical examination that they have learned in the ward is relatively uncommon in day-to-day practice. The orthopaedic surgeon or the ophthalmologist, for example, focus their attention on the site of breakdown as indicated by the patient's symptoms in the context of their specialized skills. In contrast, the neurologist acts like a sleuth and seeks out every smallest physical clue to help solve the patient's problem.

COMPARISON OF GENERAL AND HOSPITAL PRACTICE

In general practice doctors see patients in quick succession, each presenting problems demanding different clinical skills. In a single morning they might use the special skills of the gynaecologist, the ophthalmologist, the surgeon and the neurologist, in identifying the needs of their patients. The relative importance of the different skills needed in general practice is shown in Table 6.1, which

Table 6.1. The number and percentage of consultations in 1 year—analysed into 20 diagnostic groups based on the RCGP classification

Diagnostic groups	Number of consultations	Percentage
Communicable diseases	551	2.61
Neoplasms	353	1.67
Allergic, endocrine, metabolic, and nutritional diseases	866	4.11
Diseases of blood and blood-forming organs	289	1.37
Mental, psychoneurotic, and personality disorders	2534	12.01
Diseases of the nervous system	581	2.75
Diseases of the eyes	343	1.63
Diseases of the ear	607	2.88
Diseases of the circulatory system	1414	6.70
Diseases of the respiratory system (acute)	4140	19.63
Diseases of the respiratory system (chronic)	1173	5.56
Diseases of the digestive system	1656	7.58
Diseases of the genito-urinary system	928	4.40
Deliveries and complications of pregnancy, childbirth, and puerperium	344	1.63
Diseases of skin and cellular tissue	1462	6.93
Diseases of bones and organs of movement	1450	6.87
Congenital malformation and certain diseases of early infancy	44	0.21
Symptoms and ill-defined conditions	266	1.26
Accidents, poisoning, and violence	1075	5.10
Prophylactic and administrative procedures	1018	4.83
Total	21 094	100.00

separates the number and percentage of consultations in one practice during one year into different diagnostic categories. Acute respiratory disease is clearly the most common cause of a consultation in general practice, accounting for nearly 20 per cent of consultations. It is followed by mental illness (12 per cent), digestive disorders (8 per cent), and diseases of the skin (7 per cent).

In any system of medical care that makes care accessible to all individuals, irrespective of their economic resources, primary physicians will be forced to limit the time made available for each patient. When access is easy, the threshold of symptoms leading to a demand for care is likely to be lower than when access is more difficult. As a result, the probability of a patient's symptoms indicating serious disease is likely to be smaller, and the pressure on the doctor to reach an immediate diagnosis might be less. In many cases the doctor can allow the disease to pursue its natural history, confident that the patient has easy access should the disease take an unexpected course. In making an assessment of the patient's needs for medical care, the general practitioner is therefore in a very different situation to the hospital specialist. The patient who attends the specialist has been selected to do so by the general practitioner and thus the probability of such a patient having significant disease is much greater. In addition, the specialist is expected to make a diagnosis on the basis of one or two consultations and is unable to provide the easy access characteristic of the primary physician. The degree of selection that takes place when referring from generalist to specialist varies for different groups of diseases and is shown in Table 6.2. This shows, for example, that those groups of diseases that cause the greatest number of consultations in general practice, such as acute respiratory diseases and mental illness, are rarely referred to the hospital out-patient department.

Table 6.2. Outpatient referral rates per 1000 consultations for different disease groups

Diagnostic groups	Patient referral rate per 1000 consultations
Neoplasms	70
Disease of the digestive system	34
Diseases of bone and organs of movement	32
Accidents, poisoning, and violence	29
Diseases of circulatory system	23
Diseases of skin	16
Mental illness	11
Chronic respiratory disease	10
Acute respiratory disease	7
All consultations	21

The low referral rate for these contrasting groups of diseases illustrates another important aspect of general practitioners' work. In cases of acute respiratory illness they are dealing with diseases that are largely self-limiting. In those that do not fit into this category, for example, acute bronchitis and pneumonia, they have drugs available that will rapidly terminate the illness. Thus patients with a disease from this category will either get better spontaneously or will be cured by the doctor. In contrast, patients with mental illnesses seen in general practice have problems that are largely insoluble and the course of their illness is often remittent. General practitioners know that their specialist colleagues have little to offer many of these patients and recognize that they themselves are better placed to cope with their patients' illnesses. The likelihood of general practitioners referring patients to hospital, therefore, is related not only to their knowledge of the natural history of diseases but also to the probability of intervention by a specialist being able to influence the outcome of illness.

The time factor, the estimate of the probability of significant physical disease being present, and the accessibility of the general practitioner all influence the practitioner's decision to proceed from history taking to physical examination. The decision also varies with the symptoms that the patient presents. In a study that I did over a period of 1 year (Morrell *et al.* 1971) a record was kept of the presenting symptom complained of at each new consultation. An analysis of the 12 most common symptoms presented and the physical examination that took place is illustrated in Table 6.3. This again shows the importance of acquiring skills in examining the upper and lower respiratory tract and the skin. The table also illustrates the diagnostic certainty expressed by the doctors in the practice in response to different symptoms. It shows that there was no clear relationship between the extent of the physical examination of the patient and the level of diagnostic certainty recorded. Predictably, the greatest level of diagnostic certainty was recorded for symptoms that focused attention on localized areas of the body that were accessible to direct inspection.

FACILITIES

The facilities available to general practitioners that are relevant to the physical examination of their patients include those that

Table 6.3. Common symptoms analysed by the doctors diagnostic certainty and physical examination carried out expressed as percentage of total number

Symptom	Number of consultations	Diagnostic certainty		Physical examination		
		Symptomatic or provisional	Presumptive	History only	One system of the body examined	Two or more systems examined
Pain in throat	287	11	89	5	92	3
Spots and sores	182	19	81	2	97	1
Pain in ear	108	23	77	1	98	1
Cough	527	24	76	16	73	10
Pain in chest	168	51	49	1	66	33
Pain in head	159	67	33	10	57	33
Disturbance of gastric function	141	74	26	24	56	20
Pain in abdomen	197	78	21	5	60	35
Disturbance of bowel function	187	87	12	43	50	7

contribute to the best use of their time, their use of paramedical personnel, the physical conditions in which they undertake their work, and the instruments at their disposal.

During the last decade, appointment systems have become increasingly popular in British general practice and now some two-thirds of general practitioners use them. There is evidence to suggest that the introduction of an appointment system reduces the demand for services in response to acute infection and trauma, but the time made available by this fall is used by an increase in services for the elderly and the mentally ill. Studies of this subject (Morrell and Kasap 1972) showed that the introduction of an appointment system neither increased the proportion of patients examined and investigated nor reduced the proportion referred to hospital.

The premises from which general practitioners worked in the early days of the National Health Service in Britain were often inadequate. Few doctors had an examination room separate from their consulting room. It takes the average patient 4 minutes to undress and dress again. If this takes place in the general practitioner's consulting room it is time largely wasted. An examination room certainly provides an opportunity for the doctor to save time and for the patient to undress and dress in private. There is surprisingly little evidence to suggest that it increases the frequency with which doctors examine their patients.

Another major development in the British National Health Service has been the employment of nurses in the primary care situation. There is no doubt that many of the examinations and investigations that general practitioners have conventionally carried out can be undertaken equally well by nurses. This is particularly true of the continuing supervision of patients suffering from chronic diseases, for example, hypertension and diabetes. In addition, a nurse may facilitate the taking of blood and urine samples for investigation. A properly organized nursing team working closely with primary physicians does open up the possibility of doing more extensive examinations and investigations in the primary care situation.

Many books on general practice contain lists of instruments that should be kept in doctors' surgeries and bags. The contents of the surgeries will vary with the skill of the practitioners. It should be remembered that their primary function is that of diagnosticians, and if it is necessary in the interests of economy to reduce their instruments to a minimum, then they should sacrifice therapeutic for diagnostic instruments. All doctors will clearly wish to have instruments to measure a patient's weight, blood pressure, and temperature, and a diagnostic set to carry out examinations of the ear and eye. In addition, all general practitioners must possess and be able to use a vaginal speculum and proctoscope, and be able to carry out a neurological examination with a patella hammer and tuning fork. They should also have resources to collect specimens of blood, urine, sputum, stools, and for cervical cytology for laboratory investigation. Many doctors also use a microscope in the diagnosis of urinary tract infection and in other examinations, such as in skin disease and for vaginal discharges. An ECG machine is becoming increasingly common in general practice and is particularly valuable in the investigation of palpitations and chest pain. A peak flow meter is regarded as a piece of vital diagnostic equipment and is invaluable for measuring patients response to bronchodilator treatment. In all cases doctors are guided in part by the benefits to their patients as against the cost to their practice, but they might also be influenced by their special interests and the satisfaction they gain from investigating their patients more thoroughly.

WHEN TO EXAMINE

Students working in general practice will often wonder whether a physical examination is necessary to identify the patient's problem. When seeing patients, doctors should ask themselves, 'Should this patient be examined and if so, what should be the extent of the examination?' Some patients clearly need examining carefully, such as people complaining of abdominal pain or bleeding, but others do not, such as those merely seeking information. Between these extremes are large numbers of people complaining of symptoms that could be indicative of serious disease, but which usually indicate only minor abnormalities.

During the winter a doctor might, in the course of a day, encounter 10 people complaining of cough. A full examination of the upper and lower respiratory tracts will take 5–10 minutes for each patient, and therefore nearly 1½ hours a day would be spent doing such examinations, which might be totally unproductive. The doctor must therefore try to select patients who require a full examination from those suffering from only a mild, upper respiratory infection who can be dealt with more expeditiously. In making this selection, attention will be paid to the factors mentioned in history-taking. Knowing the patient's previous health record, the sort of person he or she is, and how quickly he or she seeks medical aid, is often of great value. The appearance of the patient, a history of pyrexia or malaise, listening to the cough, noting any signs of dyspnoea, and the characteristics of the sputum, will all give some indication of the seriousness of the situation. A decision may then be made whether further examination is required or whether simple advice or symptomatic treatment will suffice.

COMMON SYMPTOMS

Many symptoms are common in general practice, for example, headache, backache, nasal catarrh, indigestion, and a host of others. Any of them can indicate serious disease but generally they do not. In dealing with them it is important to develop a sense of balance and certain observations are relevant to this:

1. A symptom of recent onset, occurring in a patient who is not obviously ill and therefore alert, moving about easily, and apyrexial is unlikely to indicate serious acute infection.

2. General practitioners are in close contact with their patients, and know which ones can be trusted to return if requested to do so. In the management of these patients doctors are unlikely to lose anything by advising symptomatic treatment and then, if they do not get better, reviewing the situation.

3. Treatment of this sort must be limited to the use of simple drugs for the relief of symptoms, for example, aspirin for pain, linctus codeine for cough, and kaolin mixture for diarrhoea. To use more powerful drugs, such as antibiotics, hormones, or diuretics in this way, before making a definite diagnosis, is dangerous.

These examples are considered in more detail later but they are mentioned at this point to show that it is often safe and economic to provide advice on symptomatic treatment without conducting a full examination of the patient.

IDENTIFYING PROBLEMS

Time devoted to good history-taking will indicate the kind of abnormality that should be sought thus saving time in the examination. It is impossible to consider the type of examination that should be conducted for all the common symptoms, but all doctors should have routines that they have prepared, and which with practise, they can conduct quickly without missing any of the essentials. These routines will not be the same as those carried out by hospital specialists who deal with a very select group of individuals, but they will be devised as methods for screening all the 'suspects' so that when abnormalities are detected, more detailed examinations may be conducted.

In carrying out this examination, it is important to know what to look for and this will depend on the history-taking. It is equally important not to waste time in discursive history-taking in an attempt to avoid examination. If in doubt about whether to examine the patient, the quickest way is to proceed at once with examination. Some examples might help to clarify the type of approach used by general practitioners.

UPPER RESPIRATORY INFECTION

A patient might present complaining of nasal obstruction or 'catarrh', sore throat, and feeling unwell. This might or might not be accompanied by a cough. This is a common presenting syndrome. The questions that the doctor must try to answer by an examination are: should this patient be in bed?; is time off work necessary?; will treatment with simple symptomatic remedies suffice, or are antibiotics indicated? The answers to these questions will depend on examination findings and the abnormalities that will be sought are evidence of fever, purulent nasal discharge, infected tonsils, inflamed tympanic membrane, and lymphadenopathy. This examination can be completed in about 3 minutes. Frequently no abnormality is detected and the doctor will depend on the history for the diagnosis and treatment. By adopting this routine, however, patients can be screened for significant infection and when detected, the doctor will be in a position to treat it energetically and early, which will save not only the patient's time but also the doctor's time.

COUGH

Many patients consult their doctor complaining of cough, particularly during the winter. From the history they can be divided into those who are suffering from an acute infection of recent onset and those in whom the cough has been present for some time or has become worse recently but is essentially chronic in nature. These are treated differently with regards to examination.

Many patients complaining of cough during the winter months are suffering from upper respiratory infections. Others have minor inflammatory conditions of the lower respiratory tract, which initially produce some inflammatory hyperaemia followed by excessive mucous secretion. These present with a dry painful cough that subsequently becomes more productive with relief of pain. The question that the doctor has to answer by an examination is whether this is the onset of a more serious disorder such as bronchitis or even pneumonia. In this case it will be important to recognize the signs of toxaemia, to look for pyrexia and dyspnoea, and to inspect the sputum.

If a patient is obviously ill, a careful examination of the chest is essential. If a patient is not ill, a decision has to be made whether the illness will respond to simple symptomatic remedies or whether it demands specific antibacterial treatment. In this situation, examination will be directed to the upper respiratory tract to look for signs of a purulent discharge from the sinuses or its presence in the post-nasal space, and auscultation of the chest for signs of bronchitis, pneumonia, or cardiac failure.

In patients presenting with a cough of some weeks duration, the doctor's approach will be somewhat different. The group will include a number who are well known as chronic bronchitics and an enquiry about the colour of the sputum might be all that is required to determine the necessity for antibiotic treatment. The patient who presents for the first time, however, with a cough of some weeks duration must be submitted to a full clinical examination of the chest and cardiovascular system and a chest X-ray.

ABDOMINAL PAIN

This is another common presenting symptom that can be conveniently considered under the headings of acute or chronic disease. Abdominal pain of recent onset (hours or days) is one of the
few conditions in general practice that really demands immediate
attention. Once again the initial examination will be directed to
determine the presence or absence of fever in an attempt to decide
whether this is acute inflammatory disease. Even in the absence of
systemic signs, the doctor will proceed to examination of the
abdomen as acute inflammation may be present without systemic
upset. If there are no signs of peritoneal irritation, attention will
then be directed to the possibility of obstruction in the bowel, the
ureters, or the bile duct, etc., or to torsion of some mobile viscus,
and finally to lesions in the abdominal wall. If the patient is
obviously ill but has no localizing signs in the abdomen, examination must proceed to the lungs and throat. Particularly in
children, tonsillitis or pneumonia may present with abdominal
pain, and this becomes highly probable when the pyrexia is out of
all proportion to the abnormal signs detected on examination of
the abdomen.

In a symptom of this type when examination is mandatory, there
is a risk of skimping history-taking to get on with the examination
in the hope of making a quick diagnosis. This might be justified
when the first few sentences of the history indicate a diagnosis of
appendicitis, but because the history is usually so much more
informative than examination in the early diagnosis of intra-
abdominal disease, the 'quick up on the couch, hand on the
abdomen', approach will lead to a lot of misdiagnosis. In abdominal pain of a less acute nature, the history is all-important and
clinical examination is usually, at the most, confirmatory of a
provisional diagnosis. In many of these cases the need for radiological examination must be considered. An enormous quantity of
barium is poured unnecessarily into a variety of orifices and therefore it is important to frame the question that this further investigation is expected to answer beforehand.

With the recent technical advances in endoscopy, referral to an
endoscopy unit before carrying out barium studies might be less
traumatic for the patient and give the answer more quickly. In

addition, ultrasound is becoming increasingly valuable in the diagnosis of abdominal pain.

HEADACHE

This is one of the most difficult symptoms for the general practitioner to assess. The textbook descriptions of headache and their pathological significance are so rarely relevant to the patients who consult the general practitioner complaining of headache that they are almost valueless. Raised intracranial pressure, meningeal irritation, and hypertension are very rarely the cause of headache in general practice but figure prominently in the textbook.

There is no doubt that one of the commonest causes of headache is the pyrexia and toxaemia caused by acute infection, particularly affecting the upper respiratory tract. Attention will therefore initially be directed to answering the question, 'Has the patient an acute infection?' If the answer is 'Yes', this infection must be localized and treated in its own right. Rarely the infection will indeed involve the meninges, but it is the degree of incapacity of the patient rather than the symptom of headache that will direct the doctor to look for signs of meningitis.

In the absence of infection, headaches will either be chronic and recurrent, or very rarely acute and dramatic in onset. In an intracranial catastrophe such as subarachnoid haemorrhage, the patient will almost invariably lie still and be frightened to move compared with the hysterical outburst, when the patient rolls about holding the head and shouting with anguish. The necessity for full examination in these cases will be self-evident. It is in dealing with chronic recurrent headache that the doctor might be more confused about the extent and direction of the examination.

History-taking is again all-important, and indeed with disorders such as migraine, physical examination will add nothing of value to the diagnosis. There remain, however, some patients who do not fit into any such classical syndrome and in some of them an emotional basis might be suspected. Here it is useful to have a short examination procedure that will help clarify the situation. This might start with an inspection of the optic fundi to exclude retinopathy or papilloedema, and might be followed by a test of visual acuity. This is particularly valuable in the elderly when a significant deterioration of visual acuity might indicate glaucoma, and in all groups, any gross visual loss may be relevant. In the course of ophthalmoscopy the pupillary reactions should also be examined. Attention might then be directed to the upper respiratory tract where chronic infection may be an aetiological factor. The cervical spine might then come in for scrutiny when neck movement might be tested. Then there is the question of blood pressure. Only rarely is hypertension a cause of headache, but because the public associate headaches with high blood pressure it is essential, for the patient's peace of mind, for it to be measured. Unless some gross abnormality is detected, the patient should be firmly reassured and this in itself might produce a complete cessation of headaches. This short examination will take only about 5 minutes; its diagnostic value probably being less than its therapeutic value. Even when the doctor is certain from the history that the patient's illness is mental rather than physical, this brief examination allows both doctor and patient to proceed, if desired, to a deeper evaluation of the emotional factors involved with mutual confidence.

BACKACHE

There can be few symptoms about which there is more ignorance, in terms of pathogenesis, then backache. It is a happy hunting ground for theorists, and though one doctor might treat a patient with complete bed rest, another might treat the same patient with violent manipulation. The questions that have to be answered by physical examination therefore depend on the doctor's preconceived ideas about the aetiology of backache.

When a patient presents with backache of dramatically acute onset, occurring while lifting or adopting some unusual posture, it will be safe to say that some acute mechanical derangement of the spine has probably occurred. This might produce local pain, with accompanying rigidity of the spine and protective muscle spasm, or it might produce signs of nerve root compression. Examination will therefore be directed to clarifying this differential diagnosis and will include the demonstration of limitation of movement, muscle spasm, usually in the absence of local tenderness, and the presence or absence of signs of nerve root compression, such as pain on straight leg raising and alteration of reflexes or sensation.

Pain of less acute onset and chronic backache are notoriously difficult symptoms to assess. If present for less than a week and unaccompanied by constitutional upset, examination might be limited to an assessment of spinal movements and palpation for local tenderness, after which symptomatic treatment might be justified for a few days. The object here will be to estimate the degree of incapacity and the possible value of symptomatic treatment. Chronic recurrent backache, or backache becoming progressively worse over a period of weeks, will demand a full examination of the back, legs, and abdomen and, in many cases, pelvic examination and examination of the urine. It will often be necessary to supplement this with radiological assessment and haematology. The history will be particularly important. Chronic degenerative disease of the spinal joints is very common and it is easy to blame a few harmless osteophytes for symptoms, the origin of which might be located more accurately in the mind.

VAGUE SYMPTOMS

It is common in general practice to be faced with a patient who complains of feeling vaguely unwell, 'run down', always tired or in need of a tonic. It is tempting, in the middle of a busy surgery, to provide the tonic or a few iron tablets and proceed with the next patient. It would seem that the alternative is to take a full history and carry out a complete physical overhaul. In managing this symptom the doctor will make full use of previously acquired knowledge about the patient. These patients may be conveniently divided into three groups. There are those who are always run down, tired, or depressed, many of whom for very good reasons that might be mental, social, or physical. At some time they should be fully assessed. They tend to recur and need the doctor's sympathy or encouragement, sometimes symbolized in a prescription. The second group consists of patients who take longer than usual to recover from acute illnesses, some of whom regard the prescription of a 'tonic' as the natural sequel to specific treatment. Finally, there is a group of patients who do not commonly consult the doctor and who present with these vague symptoms.

When assessing this symptom, doctors should therefore try to decide what sort of people they are dealing with and if patients come into the third group, they should carry out full clinical examinations. The desirability of this has been confirmed by studies that have recorded the frequency with which serious illness is detected in this group. In a small series of cases, depression was the commonest diagnosis, but anaemia (including two cases with a haemoglobin below 7 grams per 100 ml) myxoedema, carcinoma of the cervix, and tuberculosis, all presented in this way. In the absence of mental illness, an abnormality might have to be sought fairly vigorously and examination will often entail the use of radiological and pathological services.

Case 38. Mrs R. came to the doctor asking for a tonic. She said she had felt 'run down' for some weeks. Only on questioning did she admit that she felt a little breathless on exertion. Physical examination disclosed no abnormality except a suspicion of anaemia. Haemoglobinometry, however, showed that she was severely anaemic (Hb 6 grams per 100 ml). Full haematological examination disclosed a hypochromic anaemia. It was only on further questioning that she admitted to menorrhagia, which she had previously regarded as normal 'at her time of life'.

EVALUATION OF COMMON SYMPTOMS OF ILLNESS

These few examples have been included, not with any claim that they represent the ideal or the only way of determining the appropriate method of examination, but to portray the thoughts that might determine general practitioners' approach to physical examination in a field where doctors must discriminate between those patients who need more or less of their time, and to show how they try to adapt their clinical skills to the situation.

At present there is considerable ignorance about the significance of presenting symptoms in general practice, and until this is remedied by research it is difficult to decide when a patient should be regarded as a bad risk and submitted to thorough investigation. There are certain symptoms, such as abdominal pain or haemorrhage, that are universally regarded as highly significant, but with many symptoms general practitioners depend as much on their previous knowledge of patients as on the complaints with which they are presented. It is difficult and dangerous to lay down hard and fast rules but the following guidelines might be helpful:

1. A full examination should always be carried out when a patient of previously stable personality presents a vague symptom. The more vague the presenting symptom, for example, loss of energy or loss of appetite, the more significant it will usually be. The reason for this is the difficulty that such patients experience in presenting the doctor with apparently trivial symptoms. A patient will often wait months before complaining of loss of appetite, but will report at once with pain in the chest.

2. If somatic symptoms are thought to be due to mental illness, physical examination is usually essential. It is difficult to convince a patient that his headache is due to anxiety until he feels that, by examination, the doctor has excluded organic disease. In addition, acute infections or endocrine imbalance will often produce mental disturbance, particularly in the elderly.

3. The presence of weight loss or persistent pyrexia should raise a very strong suspicion of the presence of a serious organic disorder. In general practice these measurements are not carried out as a matter of routine. When there is doubt about the significance of symptoms, it is often valuable to institute regular weighing and to provide patients with thermometers and temperature charts to record their temperatures. This will often help to resolve problems in which clinical examination has failed to show any abnormality.

4. Patients who are regular attenders at the surgery or on the chronic visiting list should be fully examined at least once a year. In those who are suffering from chronic disease, it is very easy to repeat a prescription regularly without considering the nature of the illness, which is essentially a dynamic and not a static condition. If the problem is thoroughly reviewed at intervals, the risk of continuing to prescribe drugs that have long since become unnecessary, or of failing to deal with some new development, will be avoided.

5. The patient's relatives are often valuable in assessing the significance of symptoms and the necessity for full examination. Some people tend to belittle their symptoms. 'A touch of rheumatism', which the doctor might dismiss may, in fact, be backache that is interfering with the whole household, and indeed sometimes the

office or workshop. A word with a wife or mother may often indicate the seriousness of a situation that was previously unsuspected (case 28).

AIDS TO DIAGNOSIS

Most of the problems encountered in general practice can be solved by careful history-taking, supported when necessary by physical examination. In a minority of cases, however, laboratory or X-ray investigations are required. Nearly all general practitioners now have access to hospital laboratory and X-ray departments and can, if they wish, ask the advice of pathologists or radiologists, or request domiciliary consultations. In using these services it is important for doctors to decide how the information obtained will help them make their diagnoses. When in doubt it is often tempting to play for time by carrying out investigations. This is rarely justified. The resources are expensive and general practitioners should always carefully consider the questions that they are asking them to answer. Intelligent use of laboratory services demands continuing education about the tests available and the significance of the results provided. Students who are accustomed to the profligate use of laboratory and X-ray investigations might reflect the impact of such an approach by general practitioners on the resources available.

Some laboratory tests are suitable for use in the doctor's consulting room and in recent years great progress has been made in developing quick and simple tests. A range of easily interpreted and reliable tests for abnormal constituents in the urine have been produced. Similar tests have been developed for detecting blood in the faeces, and there is no reason why this should not be carried out routinely at every rectal examination thus greatly extending the value of this examination.

A common condition in general practice is urinary infection. There is no doubt that bacteriological examination of a mid-stream specimen of urine is desirable for the proper treatment of this condition. It is not, however, always possible, such as in the differential diagnosis of abdominal pain or vomiting, when a result is required at once. If the doctor possesses a microscope and uses a standard method of examining urine, results can be obtained that correlate closely with more refined methods. The sight of masses of pus cells might not indicate the type of infection present, but it is very reassuring diagnostically when faced with an ill patient. The introduction of the 'dip slide' has greatly facilitated the bacteriological examination of urine.

The detection of anaemia at an early stage, before specific symptoms have developed, will enable the doctor to relieve some complaints of vague ill-health. In the past the big objection to this has been the expense of quick and accurate haemoglobinometers. Some progress has been made recently in this field and there are now several machines on the market. Accuracy to plus or minus 10 per cent is sufficient for screening purposes and a more accurate value may then be determined by the pathologist. Measurement of blood sugar can be carried out accurately in general practice, and many companies are now introducing autoanalysers of blood chemistry and plasma cholesterol for use by general practitioners. In specialized laboratories such equipment is subject to repeated validation and the mass production of such equipment, unless supported by regular audit, may give unreliable results.

In many ways general practitioners are at an advantage over their hospital colleagues in that they are not called on to provide the diagnosis at one consultation. Specialists see patients and endeavour to carry out all necessary investigations before expressing their opinion. Inevitably this may sometimes lead to the ordering of a whole battery of tests in the hope of obtaining all the information required. General practitioners are much better placed to work their way through problems. This might demand several consultations, but at each they will learn more about their patients and will know which questions need answering.

The problem of whether to obtain specimens for bacteriological culture before using antibiotics often worries students. The counsels of perfection regarding this problem, which might be simple to follow in hospital, are often impossible to follow in domiciliary practice. The time required for collection, labelling, and transport of specimens is prohibitive and furthermore the strain that this would impose on the laboratories would cause a breakdown in the services. As with other laboratory tests, it is necessary to decide to what extent the bacteriologist will help in diagnosis and treatment. In most acute infections doctors will proceed with antibiotic treatment on the basis of probability, only resorting to bacteriology when the response is unsatisfactory.

EXAMINATION OF CHILDREN

Doctors' reputations are made perhaps more by their management of children than by any other factor. If they are to be successful with children, they must like them and know how to make them like doctors. This is something students should be able to learn in general practice.

Up to the age of 1 year, most babies are not very discriminating and success is often achieved more by luck than by good judgement. The things that will most disturb a baby of this age are sudden movement and sudden noises. The doctor's approach must therefore be by stealth. Time given to history taking, during which the baby can become used to the doctor's presence, is always well invested. Examination may then proceed, preferably from the periphery as most babies will tolerate, or even enjoy, having their hands or feet played with. Examination of the abdomen will most easily be accomplished with the baby held over the mother's shoulder in the position adopted for 'winding'. To lie a baby on it's back is to court disaster.

Examination of the chest may be done after ascertaining that the stethoscope is warm. When examining the ears the baby should be sitting up and held against the mother's bosom in such a way that it can see what is going on. The light of the auroscope often provides some amusement prior to the inspection of the tympanic membranes. It is difficult to achieve examination of the throat without tears. If crying occurs early in examination, it often provides an ideal opportunity to take a quick look at the throat.

At the age of 18 months children become shy of strangers and this may persist up to the age of about 3 years. Thereafter most family doctors will be completely accepted by the child. This age group is therefore the most difficult to examine. The shy child is best ignored until it makes an approach on its own. Mothers should be encouraged to bring the baby when consulting the doctor themselves or better still with older children. When a child has left the surgery unmolested on two or three occasions it will generally be ready to submit to examination. The antenatal attendance is a particularly good time to introduce children to the doctor and to the pregnancy. If an older brother or sister is visiting the doctor, a baby will gain great confidence by seeing the older child examined and it is often possible to make the examination into something of a game.

If the child is a stranger to the doctor, the approach must be very slow. The mother should be deterred from presenting the child to the doctor and instead should present herself leaving the child free to investigate the situation. The doctor should always remain seated and when entering a child's home or bedroom should sit down as soon as possible in the deepest armchair. In this way the doctor will blend with the surroundings and present less of a threat to the child. With patience most children will accept doctors, but it is with this age group that they are most likely to have their failures. They should never use threats or force and should not allow the parents to do so. The secret is to use every contact with the child as an opportunity to build up goodwill so that an easy relationship will have already been established before the child becomes ill.

From the age of 4 years most children will submit to examination without trouble, but honesty is essential. To say 'This will not hurt' and then stick a needle into a child is asking for trouble in the future. To say that it will hurt, carry out the same procedure, and reward the child with a sweet will do little permanent damage.

The doctor's relationship with the children in his or her practice should be something that grows from the very first visit when the child is brought, often at the time of the mother's postnatal examination. The more the doctor can see the child during the ensuing months, the easier will his or her task become, not only in examining the child but in assessing the significance of any findings, and it is through the child that the doctor reaches the mother and in time, the whole family.

REFERENCES

Morrell, D., Gage, H., and Robinson, N. (1971). Symptoms in general practice. *Journal of the Royal College of General Practitioners*, **21**, 32–43.

Morrell, D. and Kasap, K. (1972). Effect of an appointment system on demand for medical care. *International Journal of Epidemiology*, **1**, 143–51.

7

Prognosis

Although diagnostic competence is the most vital skill for good general practitioners to acquire, their reputation depends on the art of prognosis. Patients might be interested to know the diagnosis, but usually this means very little to them and it is prognosis that is more important to them. Often this function is given only scant attention in the training of a doctor.

What doctors say to patients in particular situations plays a big part in general practitioners' lives. They depend on their ability to prognosticate when issuing certificates and when planning visits and surgery consultations. Success will be reflected in a smooth running practice whereas failure will result in a hectic life interspersed with avoidable emergencies.

Case 39. Mrs M. came to the doctor complaining of a rash on her chest and pain. The doctor told her that she had shingles and advised local treatment, but 2 days later was called at 10pm because Mrs M. was in severe pain. The doctor prescribed analgesia, and 5 days later was called again because the pain was not better. Mrs M. was extremely displeased and depressed.

In this case the diagnosis was correct, but the doctor failed to appreciate the amount of pain Mrs M. would suffer and failed to impress on her the implications of the diagnosis. Had she been told to expect pain for 3–4 weeks, been prescribed adequate analgesia, and arrangements made to see her again to support her during the illness, the doctor would have had a happier patient and fewer emergency calls.

Case 40. Mr R. also complained of a rash on his chest. The doctor correctly diagnosed pityriasis rosea and explained that it was not serious and that there was no treatment. Two weeks later Mr R. came back asking indignantly for an appointment with a skin specialist. The doctor was annoyed at this request and endeavoured unsuccessfully to point out that this was quite unnecessary.

Once again the diagnosis was correct but the prognosis had not been fully explained to the patient. Had the doctor told Mr R. that the rash was harmless but would persist for 3–5 weeks, and suggested that he should visit the surgery in 2 weeks time so that he could be checked to see that all was well, Mr R. would have concluded that he had a clever and attentive doctor.

These are simple examples, but they reflect the influence of prognostic accuracy on the doctor-patient relationship, and on the use of the doctor's time. In planning revisits and surgery consultations, it is important to be able to predict the probable course of events in any individual case. It is usually not difficult to assess the success that is achieved in this direction. If doctors are being too cautious they will find that they are doing a lot of unnecessary consultations. If, on the other hand, they err in the opposite direction, they will find themselves recalled to patients whom they had seen a few days before, and will probably also have a large number of emergency calls.

The descriptive accounts of prognosis in medical textbooks give the impression that it depends entirely on the diagnosis. It does, however, more than any other aspect of medicine, depend on the individual. When considering prognosis the doctor must make a complete diagnosis, relating the pathology present to the individual concerned. Even when an accurate diagnosis is made, it can be notoriously difficult to predict the course of events in a given instance of a disease. In general practice the diagnosis is often in doubt, at least in the early stages, and this further complicates the task.

In addition, prognosis as described in textbooks is often derived from information collected from the highly selected population of patients who attend hospital. Very few studies of the natural history of disease have been carried out in general practice. Those that have been done often disclose facts that are at variance with traditional teaching. These facts are important to the general practitioner in making a prognosis.

In his valuable book *Common diseases: their nature, incidence, and care*, Fry (1974) described the natural history of many of the common diseases seen in general practice. On the basis of data collected over a period of 25 years he showed; for example, that a peptic ulcer first diagnosed in general practice has a comparatively good prognosis with a 60 per cent rate of spontaneous recovery.

He also described the outcome of illnesses not seen in hospital, such as the prolonged period of malaise and depression that may follow influenza. While working in general practice doctors can slowly accumulate this type of knowledge, but they now have the advantage of a synthesis of information painstakingly acquired by workers such as Fry.

FACTORS INFLUENCING PROGNOSIS

The most obvious factors affecting prognosis are the physical characteristics of the individual. Of these, age is probably the most important. The elderly respond to acute traumatic incidents poorly, and the healing of fractures is notoriously difficult to predict in this age group. In the infant it might be hazardous to give a prognosis because illnesses such as measles, whooping cough, and pneumonia in children under the age of 2 years are still serious diseases. Older children can be equally alarming to their parents, developing high fevers, often in response to quite minor infections. They are, however, very resilient and within 24 hours a seriously ill child may be demanding a normal diet and racing round the house. The progress of certain diseases, such as cancer and hypertension, is closely related to age, being more aggressive in the young adult than in the elderly.

The nutrition of the patient should be considered when making a prognosis. In the absence of some abnormality of absorption, malnutrition is rarely seen nowadays except in old people. It almost certainly reduces the patient's resistance to infection and delays healing. Obesity is more common and has an adverse effect on patients suffering from conditions such as osteoarthritis and cardiac failure, although it offers a remedial cause for the symptoms. In this case the prognosis will be related to the patient's ability to lose weight.

The presence of chronic disorders will influence the individual's response to new acute episodes of illness. The poor response of the diabetic or the steroid-dependent patient to acute infection and pulmonary tuberculosis is well known. Acute respiratory infection carries particular hazards for the chronic bronchitic, the asthmatic, for patients suffering from cardiac failure, and for a variety of other disorders. Patients suffering from osteoarthritis, venous thrombosis, or simple old age are likely to deteriorate if they develop an illness that demands bed rest.

These are just a few examples of the way in which diseases might interact, and in framing their prognoses doctors should always consider the relevance of any preceding illness to the current disease.

Any disturbance of mental health will also influence prognosis. This is much less clearly defined, but it is well known that, aside from physique, some patients are able to tolerate ill health far better than others. This might be partly a question of pain threshold, but some patients have a resilience that allows them to pursue a normal life despite marked infirmity. At the opposite extreme, there are patients in every practice who find it necessary to seek medical aid for every minor disturbance. This mental determination to survive may affect prognosis in both directions. It is usually a good sign, but occasionally individuals drive themselves beyond their physical or mental capabilities thus causing them to completely collapse.

It is well recognized that widows and widowers are more likely to die in the year following the loss of their marital partner than are other individuals of the same age and sex. They are also more likely to suffer physical illness and to make demands on their general practitioner (Levy 1976).

In certain individuals, physical illness may swing the balance to produce frank depression or mania and conversely mental illness may occasionally lead to physical breakdown. These complex factors all have to be considered when making a prognosis, but often they scarcely reach consciousness and are reflected in the doctor's remarks, for example, 'He will be over that in a day or two and back to work', or alternatvely 'He always needs a week off when he gets a cold'. Doctors know that patients respond to situations in particular ways, but they would find it difficult to say why. These characteristics are often reflected in patients' medical records.

Careful studies of depression (Brown *et al.* 1975) have shown that several social factors determine whether an individual reacts to a serious life event by becoming depressed. Thus a woman is more likely to become depressed if she lost her own mother before the age of 11 years, if she has no intimate confidant (husband or boyfriend), if she has three or more children under the age of 15 years, or if she is unemployed. This elegant research provides information that helps general practitioners to identify those patients who are particularly vulnerable to mental illness.

Social factors are perhaps more easily understood than mental factors. The need for money often drives a man to work when he is unfit for it, and the needs of her children keep a woman at the kitchen sink when she would be better off in bed. With minor ailments this need to get better improves the prognosis, but in more serious illness it can impede treatment and recovery.

The patient's home conditions will influence the rate of recovery in many instances. Overcrowding and lack of proper washing facilities render the treatment of conditions such as impetigo and other skin diseases most difficult, and the excellent prognosis that might be given in a well-provided home must be modified. If housing is very poor, patients who could normally be treated at home might require hospital treatment. The presence of a competent mother and father will facilitate the recovery of children whereas a house full of children may worsen mother's prospects if she falls ill. The opportunity to summon the aid of relatives or neighbours during convalescence leads to a more satisfactory outcome than can be expected when a person has to leave a sick-bed and fend for him or herself.

In the elderly, the site of the dwelling may affect the patient's return to health. The presence of stairs or hills, or the paucity of local shops or public transport, will tend to isolate those who suffer from heart disease, chronic bronchitis, or arthritis. Occupation should always be carefully considered when telling patients how long they are likely to be off work. Repair of a hernia in a 'navvy' will require a more prolonged period off work than the same operation in an office worker. Doctors in hospital often tend to underestimate the effect of operative treatment. Patients leave hospital apparently fit 5 days after an appendicectomy, and it is not until doctors enter general practice that they realize that such patients are far from fit at this stage and will need another 3–4 weeks off work to convalesce.

The ability to assess how any given individual will respond to illness comes only after observing that person in health, in disease, and in the context of his or her family and work. After working in a practice for many years doctors will usually become expert in dealing with their own patients. The importance of this knowledge can be confirmed by any doctors who have changed from one practice to another and noticed how poor their performances become when faced with new communities. To some extent this can be offset by good record-keeping; well-kept notes should reflect far more than a list of the diseases from which the patient has suffered. They should provide a thumb-nail sketch of the individual's behaviour in response to illness.

Having considered all these factors and decided on the prognosis, the doctor is then in a position to tell the patient the conclusions thus reached. It must, however, be emphasized that these conclusions are based on knowledge that is often limited and on interpretation of disease, which is liable to error. The doctor should therefore beware of pontifical statements and of using the words 'always' and 'never'. How much should be said in cases of serious illness is a subject of constant debate and, before giving any firm advice on this matter, it is worth mentioning some general considerations.

1. The contract between a doctor and patient is such that the patient has a right, in justice, to the truth. This right is perfectly clear in private practice when the patient pays directly for the consultation. There is, however, a tendency to forget that precisely the same relationship exists with patients who pay their doctor through insurance contributions and taxation.

2. The doctor has a duty to his patient '...to comfort always'.

3. In the family doctor–patient relationship, the doctor also has a duty to other members of the family. If the doctor comforts grandad with a lot of lies, will the rest of the family ever be able to trust him or her in the future?

In the simple everyday problems of practice these duties rarely cause conflict. It is in serious and fatal illnesses that problems arise and therefore it is more profitable to consider this type of case. An extreme example is the patient who is dying from an incurable disease. The next-of-kin has been warned of this, but should the patient be told?

COMMUNICATING WITH DYING PATIENTS

Before telling patients that they are suffering from incurable disease and are likely to die, it is important to be sure that the evidence on which this prognosis is based is sound. Such a warning might seem superfluous, but the frequency with which patients boast that they have survived a fatal prognosis makes it necessary. In some cases these statements might be exaggerations of the true prognosis that was given by the doctor, but some doctors are probably a little too ready to give a bad prognosis on the basis of insufficient evidence.

Case 41. Mrs M., aged 50, developed a deep vein thrombosis and pulmonary embolus 5 years after mastectomy for cancer of the breast. She was treated with anticoagulants. Chest X-ray revealed enlarged glands in the mediastinum but a biopsy was not undertaken as she was receiving anticoagulants. She was told that she had secondary cancer in the glands of her chest and was advised of the seriousness of this situation. She was treated with local radiotherapy. She and her family became very anxious about her future. She complained of severe chest pain and began to develop panic attacks in which she became acutely breathless and expected to suffocate. She was treated with counselling, slow release morphine sulphate, and steroids. One year later her health improved and all treatment was stopped. Five years later, she is alive and well. In retrospect, it seems highly unlikely that she ever had secondary cancer in her mediastinum.

The prognosis is particularly uncertain in elderly patients suffering from cancer.

Case 42. Mr I. presented at the age of 85 with haemoptysis. Abnormal physical signs were detected in the right lung and patchy collapse distal to a mass was demonstrated on the chest X-ray. During the next 10 years, Mr I. intermittently complained of haemoptysis and had a number of chest infections. He died at the age of 95 from a cerebrovascular accident, oblivious of the fact that he had almost certainly suffered from cancer of the lung for 10 years.

The next consideration is whether the patient asks for this information. Many people who know that they are dying never ask doctors for a prognosis. This is usually out of consideration for the doctors. They know how hard it must be for doctors to tell this difficult truth and therefore wish to spare them this task. At the same time, however, they might very much want to discuss dying with them. Patients who know that the end is near often derive great comfort from discussing this with somebody. They can be reassured about relief of pain and can shed a great deal of anxiety about those that they are leaving behind. This is perhaps the most difficult kind of therapeutic listening that a doctor is ever called on to undertake, and yet by far the most rewarding. Unfortunately, too many doctors have insufficient courage to undertake this task, and rationalize their position by saying that the patient should not be told the truth.

There is another group of dying patients who ask the straight-forward question, 'Am I doing to die?', or 'Is it cancer?', which to many means the same. This presents a particular difficulty in that the question is often unexpected and yet an answer is demanded at once. The answer to this question is quite frequently in the nega-tive, but if the patient is dying it is important for the doctor to know why the patient has asked the question. In other words, the answer to this question depends on a complete diagnosis of the implications of this particular disease in this particular person. If the diagnosis is not complete a suitable rejoinder is, 'Why are you asking that question?'

For a man with a wife and several young children, it might be important for him to realize that he is dying so that he can make provision for his family. His family doctor should know whether he is asking this question in the hope of obtaining reassurance, or because he wants a truthful answer. In the latter case, he is bound in justice to tell him. Doctors very often underestimate the cour-age of patients and it is sometimes a comfort to the doctor to remember that men are prepared to face almost certain death for their country in war, and most would be happy to sacrifice more for their wife and family.

The question of religion must also be considered. Christians, Moslems, Jews, among others, for example believe that life on earth is but a preparation for a life after death. To them dying is a very important event and one for which they wish to prepare. Many pray to be protected from sudden and unprepared death. Doctors who have no religious convictions themselves might find it difficult to understand this philosophy of life but they have no right to ignore it. It is the highest form of charity to warn such a person of impending death, and doctors should not let their own weak-nesses or unbelief prevent them from fulfilling their duty in this direction.

Finally there are the people who occupy important posts in public life. These people, in taking high office, are accepting serious responsibilities that carry with them duties to the community.

It is often necessary for them to be made fully aware of the implications of their disease.

These remarks will illustrate that there is no easy answer to the question, 'Should the doctor tell?'. What the doctor tells the patient is part of the treatment, and rational treatment depends on a complete diagnosis. Doctors who try to answer this question in one word are simply not facing up to their responsibilities as personal doctors. Many dying patients will say that there is no torment like the uncertainty of not knowing. No doctor has the right to deprive a patient of this comfort because he or she does not have the courage to discuss the problem frankly with the patient. Sometimes it might be best to leave the patient ignorant of impending death. This is one of the most difficult and important decisions the general practitioner is called on to make.

When, after due consideration, the doctor is not sure what to say, it is usually best to leave the patient to decide. This can be done by offering a dual prognosis. To the question, 'Am I going to die?', the doctor may answer, 'Your illness is very serious, but we hope that this treatment will help'. The patient is then at liberty to accept either the serious prognosis or the more hopeful one. The doctor must then judge whether the patient wishes to know the worst or the best, and adjust the prognosis accordingly. Patients rarely ask the direct question but tend to discuss the seriousness of the prognosis in more general terms. Here again the doctor can offer them alternatives. There appears to be some psychological mechanism by which seriously ill patients can block out the truth when they wish to avoid it, and they persist in the hope of a happy outcome despite obvious signs to the contrary. Doctors can foster this if they see it developing.

Though general practitioners are unquestionably the best people to know what is right for their patients in this situation, it is easy for them to be misled regarding this particular decision. The man with a strong personality, who thoughout life has appeared able to stand stresses and strains without apparent disturbance, might suffer more when faced with death. Having dealt so efficiently with life, he is perhaps less able to deal with the complete negation of life, over which he is impotent. It is therefore better to avoid developing preconceived ideas about the way in which any individual will react to death, and to treat each case on its merits as it progresses.

Case 43. Mr W. was aged 49 with a wife and four children. He was dying of cancer of the lung. Mr W. knew that he was dying and arranged to visit Lourdes in the hope of comfort. He came home, not cured, but very much strengthened by the experience. Mrs W. told the doctor that on no account must he tell Mr W. of the hopelessness of his prognosis. Mr and Mrs W. and the doctor all knew that the outlook was hopeless, but would not discuss the subject. Fortunately, Mr W. had a wise parish priest who succeeded in helping him in his last needs where his doctor and wife had failed.

Case 44. Mr E. was dying of secondary carcinomatosis. He explained to his doctor that he was in the habit of preparing for any big event in his life and that he regarded death as the biggest event and would appreciate plenty of notice. The doctor fell in with his wishes and during his last weeks had the pleasure of helping him by therapeutic listening and discussion, and witnessed a happy death in which Mr and Mrs E., surrounded by their family, parted company.

Case 45. Mrs C. was dying from secondary carcinomatosis. She was a simple woman with no religious beliefs. She often asked if her condition was serious, and sensing that her enquiry demanded reassurance, the doctor gave this together with adequate analgesia and she gradually drifted into unconsciousness.

'THEY NEVER TELL YOU ANYTHING'

So far, only illnesses in which the outcome is inevitably fatal have been discussed. Many of the considerations that have been mentioned also apply to less serious disease. Most people are capable of understanding the significance of death. In less serious disease it is, however, important to consider the patient's ability to comprehend the prognostic statements that the doctor might make. It is no use telling a labourer that he is suffering from a myocardial infarction, or a simple housewife that her child suffers from 'petit mal'. One of the biggest complaints levelled against hospitals is that 'They never tell you anything'. This is probably an overstatement of the facts. What the patients really mean is that they could not understand the facts that were told to them.

The art of prognosis is closely related to the ability of doctors to interpret scientific facts in language that patients can understand. It is no use talking about prolapse of the uterus when the patient can think only in terms of 'dropping of the womb'. Not only must doctors use words that the patient can understand but they must also be able to forecast the significance of these words to the individual patient. The doctor might say to a mother, 'Your child has a small patch of pneumonia', and regard this as being of little prognostic significance. The mother who thinks of pneumonia as it was thirty years ago will turn pale and demand the child's immediate admission to hospital.

This problem is therefore one that requires not only the ability to describe disease processes in simple terms but also a great sensitivity to the patients' preformed notions concerning disease. A great deal can be learned about the former by listening to experienced doctors. An effort must always be made to liken the pathological process to something with which the patient is familiar. A myocardial infarct may be likened to a cut on the skin, which heals with a scar and takes a month or two to become strong, thus emphasizing the need for rest for a few weeks. Otitis media may be likened to a boil; vaginitis to a cold in the head, which produces a discharge.

The preformed ideas of patients concerning disease can often be detected by simply asking, 'What do you think has caused this trouble?'. Patients might then volunteer their thoughts about having cancer, an ulcer, tuberculosis, or arthritis. This often gives the doctor a clue to the significance that the patient might attach to a given diagnosis, and he can frame the prognosis given accordingly. In giving a prognosis it is important to explain precisely what this means in terms of inconvenience to the patient concerned. This will often mean that the doctor must use terms that are essentially unscientific, but which are tailored to the understanding of the individual. It is wise to start by stating, as definitely as possible, whether the disease is, or is not, serious. Usually patients fear the worst and if complex dicussions are entered into before they have been reassured, they might become alarmed and fail to appreciate the problems as seen by the doctors. On rare occasions patients or relatives might seem disinterested and then it might be necessary to emphasize the seriousness of a diagnosis.

The doctor should try to be as far sighted and realistic as possible with his prognosis. It is valueless to give a good prognosis to spare the patient's feelings when the true implications of the disease will inevitably become apparent after a short time. To do so will undermine the patient's confidence in the doctor. If the prognosis is uncertain, however, it is indefensible to warn the patient of the worst possible outcome simply to safeguard the doctor from future criticism. Some examples might help to clarify this. These examples were published in the first edition of this book. Follow-up has been made possible by the co-operation of the practitioners who were responsible for the continuing care of these patients.

Case 46. Mr F. aged 28 and newly married, suffered an attack of retrobulbar neuritis with a transient visual field defect. This recovered within 2 weeks, but was thought to be the first incident in disseminated sclerosis. The doctor had to decide whether he should tell either the patient or his wife of the significance of the episode. Mr F. might never have any further trouble, or he might equally well be a cripple within 10 years. The doctor described this attack to his patient as an inflammation of the nerves that might never bother him again. He decided not to discuss the full implications of the diagnosis, and to allow Mr and Mrs F. to proceed with a normal and full married life.
Twenty five years later the doctor was telephoned by the general practitioner then concerned with the care of Mr F. The patient had just experienced his second manifestation of multiple sclerosis.

Case 47. Mr J., aged 46, developed osteoarthritis of the hip. He worked as a steel erector and, though he could manage his work despite some stiffness, his prospects of continuing in this work for many years were very poor. The doctor decided that the patient should be made aware of the implications of his diagnosis and he was encouraged to seek new employment which would not only improve his prognosis but also improve his prospects of employment in the more distant future. Twenty years later Mr J., having successfully run a newsagents in the interim period, has had a hip replacement.

Case 48. Mr M., aged 50, was a successful business man who was overweight and an excessive smoker. He was found to be suffering from hypertension. Though his life was not immediately in danger and he was symptom-free, his doctor decided that the risks involved in continuing his present mode of life were such that he must be made aware of the situation. He discussed these risks with Mr M. and was successful in persuading him to take more exercise and to eat and smoke less. During the succeeding years, Mr M.'s blood pressure was treated and he is now enjoying his retirement at the age of 68.

Case 49. Mrs H., aged 50, was overweight and also hypertensive. Because the prognosis in fat, hypertensive women is better than that in men, the doctor restricted himself to advising Mrs H. to reduce her weight. At this stage he did not feel that it was necessary to burden Mrs H. with details of her raised blood pressure. Mrs H., however, was neither able to reduce her weight nor later to comply with hypotensive treatment. She died at the age of 65 from a cerebrovascular accident.

These are but a few examples to show how the prognosis must be tailored to suit each individual and that, although what is said is based on scientific facts, the way in which this is presented reflects the doctor's proficiency in the art of medicine.

The final question that must be answered is, 'Who should be responsible for telling patients about the significance of their illnesses'?. In most cases this duty naturally falls on general practitioners as they are the only doctors involved. When hospitals are concerned there is often some uncertainty, but the ultimate responsibility, however, still rests with family doctors. They alone are fully aware of what particular disabilities mean to individuals. Doctors in hospitals might have to give patients certain information, but they are well advised to leave the interpretation of serious disease to patients' own general practitioners.

Family doctors have a continuous responsibility for their patients, which contrasts with the short-term and essentially episodic responsibility of the hospital. They should know their patients and their susceptibilities, intelligence, families, and environment far better than any consultant, whose contact is but short and often superficial. It is family doctors who will care for patients during the years to come, and it is therefore surely their privilege to say what those years might bring forth.

REFERENCES

Brown, G. and Harris, T. (1978). *Social origins of depression: a study of psychiatric disorders in women*. Tavistock, London.

Fry, J. (1979). *Common diseases: their nature, incidence, and care,* (2nd edn). Lancaster Medical and Technical Publishing Company.

Levy, R. and Balfour Sclare (1976). A study of bereavement in general practice. *Journal of the Royal College of General Practitioners*, **26,** 329–36.

8

Prevention, health education, and the primary care team

INTRODUCTION

General practitioners in the United Kingdom are responsible for defined populations of patients. If they have good records they can identify them in terms of their age, sex, address, marital state, and the major chronic diseases from which they suffer. They are therefore well placed to develop preventive and health education programmes to provide for their patients' needs. Prevention is sometimes classified into primary prevention, which is concerned with actions taken to prevent the development of disease; secondary prevention, which is concerned with identifying pre-symptomatic diseases; and tertiary prevention, which is concerned with preventing disability as a consequence of established chronic disease. Not surprisingly there is some overlap when these definitions are applied to the ongoing care in general practice.

PRIMARY PREVENTION

This covers a wide variety of initiatives that might be undertaken by general practitioners.

Immunization against disease

Primary prevention is particularly concerned with the prevention of infection by immunization. The value of this is well established and the side effects are minimal. General practitioners are uniquely placed to deliver this care, working closely with attached health visitors and practice nurses. In the course of antenatal care family doctors will establish ongoing relationships with the young mothers in their practices, which are reinforced through post-natal care and supervision of family planning. Being responsible for a defined population of patients, they can regularly audit the care provided and ensure that all those at risk are fully im-munized.

Healthy living

Children

Primary prevention extends beyond the immunization of indi-viduals against disease. It is concerned with altering patterns of human behaviour that have been shown to be detrimental to health. These include nutrition, smoking, exercise, sexual be-haviour, and the consumption of drugs and alcohol. A systematic approach aimed at identifiable 'at risk' groups may be developed in general practice as exemplified by the regular supervision of children under the age of 5 years. This is carried out by health visitors, in association with general practitioners, at 6 weeks, 7 months, 2 years, and at 3½ years.

General practitioners have access to populations of people who are in their developing years. It is well recognized that genetic factors, raised serum cholesterol, obesity, cigarette smoking, and hypertension are all associated with the development of vascular disorders. It is therefore appropriate for general practitioners to be conscious of these risks when providing care. Logically, appropriate advice about diet, such as reducing the intake of refined sugars, dairy produce, and animal fats that is given to children will be more likely to improve health than attempts to restrict the diets of middle-aged, obese men and women. General practitioners see the children in their practices four or five times a year up to the age of 7 years, and a few extra minutes devoted to health education of their parents at this stage might be more useful than hours devoted to educational programmes for the middle-aged. At the same time attention must be given to the 'at risk groups' when under-nutrition may be a problem, for example, vitamin D deficiency in Asian communities.

Adolescents

General practitioners have a major problem in the health education of the teenage population. They are likely to be seen as
authoritative figures and thus their advice might be rejected. In
dealing with this age group, they are particularly concerned with
providing advice on smoking, drugs, alcohol, and sexual promiscuity. At this stage, doctors are most likely to be asked for advice
on contraception and this is one occasion when they might have an
opportunity to intervene. Other opportunities might be presented
when consultations are made for acute respiratory illness when
smoking behaviour may be explored, or for acne when diet may be
discussed, and for gastroenterological problems, which open up
opportunities to discuss diet, alcohol, and life styles. General
practitioners have unique opportunities to promote health in the
context of their day-to-day consultations. Many of these consultations are, however, carried out in sessions restricted by serious
time constraints. Only a very positive commitment to health
promotion will ensure that the doctor accepts and takes advantage
of the opportunities presented.

The detection of obesity does not need sophisticated screening
procedures; the doctor simply needs to use his eyes. Discussion of
diet and the consumption of 'junk foods' may feature in any of the
routine consultations with parents and children. The smoking behaviour of parents is associated with the development of this habit
in children and warnings should be issued at an early age. Parental
behaviour almost certainly influences the incidence of mental illness and sexual promiscuity in adolescents and opportunities will
be presented when this can be explained to parents.

Adults

Despite the negative results in population experiments designed to
reduce the incidence of myocardial infarction, general practitioners
have a responsibility for providing advice on healthy living in
respect of this and other disorders. It has been shown that advice,
with follow-up, on smoking behaviour delivered by general practitioners does produce worthwhile results. There is good evidence
that respiratory illness in childhood, associated with parental

smoking, can produce disability from chronic respiratory disease in adult life. It is most likely that such advice will be adhered to when the individual is suffering from respiratory disability. Advice on smoking should therefore always be introduced into consultations with patients who are smokers and are currently suffering from respiratory disease.

Obesity is a cause of serious disability, particularly in those suffering from musculo-skeletal disorders. Once established it is very difficult to cure. The general practitioner must therefore give particular attention to those life events that are particularly associated with weight gain. Of these, pregnancy and childbirth are particularly important and the doctor has ample opportunities at numerous antenatal consultations to provide advice. Young adult males, particularly those in the lower social classes, are prone to gain weight that is often associated with excessive alcohol intake, and every opportunity should be taken to provide advice at a stage when this tendency can be reversed.

SECONDARY PREVENTION

This is concerned with the detection of presymptomatic disease by screening or case finding to improve the chances of medical intervention being effective. The case for multiphasic screening in general practice has been examined (The South East London Screening Study Group 1977) and it was found that in the short term, patients screened did not enjoy any more benefits than a control group in terms of morbidity, mortality, hospitalization, or sickness absence. This study also showed that almost all the patients suffering from important abnormalities were known to their general practitioners. Another study showed that all those with significantly raised blood pressure had consulted their general practitioner in the preceding 3 years (D'Souza *et al.* 1976). The concept of opportunistic case finding (Sackett and Holland 1975) then evolved as a more economical way of identifying medical need in general practice than screening. This concept is based on the fact that in the United Kingdom general practitioners see 90 per cent of their patients in 3 years, and that if they use these consultations to screen for important risk factors such as high blood pressure, they are likely to identify the majority of those needing treatment. This concept may be extended to include risk factors such as smoking, family history of coronary artery disease linked with a raised blood cholesterol, and obesity.

Infant welfare services

General practitioners and health authorities in the United Kingdom provide facilities for the routine screening of children up to the age of 5 years. This is seen as a particularly vulnerable group in the community. Routine observations of weight gain are carried out and are particularly valuable when a halt in weight gain or a loss of weight may indicate serious illness or major problems in the family. Vision, hearing, and speech development are also checked at regular intervals. More sophisticated tests of development are carried out in some clinics, but there is little evidence that they are of value in detecting illness at a presymptomatic stage when intervention will be helpful. Physical checks at these periodic medicals include examination for congenital dislocation of the hip, major cardiovascular anomalies, and abnormalities in head circumference.

Family planning

Many general practitioners are concerned with providing advice on family planning. This offers an excellent opportunity for primary prevention in giving advice on smoking, obesity, and sexual relationships. It also involves the doctor in screening a vulnerable group of individuals by regular cervical cytology, measurement of blood pressure, and instruction on breast self-examination. These consultations may also be used to confirm immunity against rubella before patients start out on a pregnancy and, if indicated, can provide opportunities for individuals to seek genetic counselling when there is a risk of inherited disorders.

Antenatal care

This is a classical example of presymptomatic screening widely practised in primary care throughout the world. Apparently healthy women are regularly monitored for signs of presymptomatic abnormalities. At the onset of pregnancy, blood tests are carried out to determine the woman's haemoglobin, blood group, rhesus state, and her immunity to rubella and to look for evidence of past infection from syphilis. At the same time the urine is screened for asymptomatic bacteruria. In selected individuals, such as mothers over the age of 36, screening for Down's syndrome may be carried out by measuring the level of alpha-fetoprotein in the blood and by performing an amniocentesis. Ultrasonography is performed at about the 16th week in pregnancy to confirm the maturity of the fetus, the position of the placenta, and to identify certain fetal abnormalities. During the pregnancy, routine observations are carried out to detect presymptomatic signs of pre-eclampsia, re-tarded fetal growth, or abnormal fetal presentations. General practitioners will also try to assess the social and family situation into which the new child will be born, and anticipate problems that might develop in the family relationship as a result of the economic consequences of the pregnancy. This preventive care extends into the immediate postnatal period. Most infants are screened for phenylketonuria and hypothyroidism in hospital following de-livery, but in some cases this responsibility devolves on the general practitioner. More importantly and routinely general practitioners are involved with observing the development of the mother–child relationship and the effect it has on family dynamics, and they have to remain aware of the possibility of emotional disorders in the mother following delivery.

Cervical cytology

Despite the fact that the link between abnormal cervical cytology and invasive carcinoma of the cervix remains tenuous, cervical screening has been widely accepted as a useful examination. Many women are introduced to cervical smears in the provision of family planning services.

General practitioners who maintain age–sex registers, either on card indexes or computers, can develop a call and recall system for cervical smears at regular intervals (3 yearly intervals are currently recommended). Practice nurses can be trained to carry out this test and in many practices this is combined with instruction on breast self-examination. There is a lot of evidence to suggest that patients prefer this examination to be carried out by someone of the same sex and the organization of cervical screening by a practice nurse is likely to lead to a higher uptake of this service. This does not, however, preclude opportunistic screening of the cervix and breasts when appropriate examinations are carried out in general practice, and this opportunistic approach may include individuals who would be unlikely to avail themselves of routine screening and who, in many surveys, have been shown to be those most at risk.

TERTIARY PREVENTION

Chronic disease

Individuals suffering from chronic degenerative disease are monitored at regular intervals in general practice. Such conditions include diabetes, hypertension, schizophrenia, chronic rheumatic disorders, and chronic vascular disorders. This usually takes the form of consultations at intervals of 1–6 months depending on the disease and the individual concerned. Structured medical records may be of special value in the provision of this type of care. Identification of groups of vulnerable patients ensures that those at risk can be immunized against influenza each winter, and that those who are housebound can be regularly visited by the doctor or the community nurse. This is the field of tertiary prevention, which aims to delay death and disability by the comprehensive and systematic care of established disease.

The elderly

Increasing numbers of people are living into their eighth and ninth decades of life. They are vulnerable to a variety of disabilities. Many general practitioners screen individuals in these age groups for disability. This screening is concerned more with the patient's ability to perform the normal functions of daily living, helped if necessary by the resources available to them for support in the community, than with the diagnosis of disease. Unfortunately, despite a more discriminating approach to the needs of the elderly it is likely that resources will continue to fail to satisfy their needs in the face of the demographic changes in society.

HEALTH PROMOTION

For decades, the consultation in general practice has been seen as the first contact for patients experiencing symptoms of illness for which they usually expect an appropriate therapeutic response, often leading to a prescription for medication. It was indeed seen as a demand led service. In a careful analysis of the content of the consultation (Morrell 1971), I showed that over half the consultations were concerned not with new episodes of illness but with the continuing care or monitoring of patients suffering from chronic disease, which is essentially tertiary prevention. Scott and Davis (1979) spelt out the potential of the consultation in general practice, which provides opportunities not only to deal with the presenting complaint but to undertake tasks concerned with health maintenance and prevention. They summarized this diagrammatically (Fig. 8.1).

Attitudes of general practitioners are slowly changing and they are beginning to appreciate the potential of their role in prevention and health promotion. One factor that might be important in determining the speed of change is the low priority with which prevention and health promotion are currently regarded in undergraduate medical education. The fact that this field of activity might be far more important in reducing disability and disease is often not stressed sufficiently to the undergraduate, and the work satisfaction and glamour that is associated with diagnostic competence and curative treatment might be overemphasized. A more realistic approach to the role of the doctor is slowly developing throughout the world. The therapeutic inadequacy of medicine in solving the problems of patients suffering from chronic degenerative diseases has led to attention being focused on the importance of prevention and the necessity to identify patients' problems, not in terms of diagnoses, but in terms of the disability produced and the resources needed in the community to reduce this disability.

This change of attitude to doctors' role in society is important. It

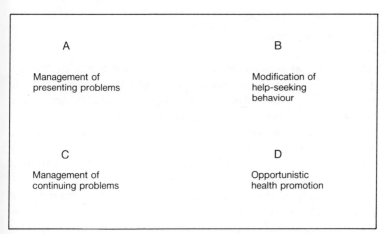

Fig. 8.1. The potential of the consultation in general practice, which can provide opportunities to deal with the presenting complaint and also with health maintenance and prevention. (From Stott, N. and Davis, R. (1979). The potential in each primary care consultation—an aide memoire. *Journal of the Royal College of General Practitioners*, **29**, 201–5.)

is necessary, however, not to emphasize this at the expense of doctors' clinical skills and therapeutic role. An overemphasis on preventive procedures and health maintenance, which might not have been properly evaluated, may distract doctors from their equally important role in responding to new symptoms of illness and may threaten their compassionate role in the community.

RESOURCES AND THE PRIMARY CARE TEAM

Primary medical, or health, care is concerned with providing health education, prevention, an appropriate response to new symptoms of illness, and the continuing care of chronic disease. It is difficult to see how one health professional can fulfil all these roles; no one person can be expected to have all the requisite knowledge and skills. In addition, if accessible to a defined community of patients they cannot be expected to have the time to provide all these services.

The nurse in primary care

Arguments put forward in favour of the nurse acting as primary diagnostician have unfortunately obscured the real role of the nurse in primary care. There are two aspects to be considered. The first is the role of the nurse in providing community nursing care. Many patients are now cared for in their own homes and here a close relationship is essential between the doctor and the nurse providing care. This is most easily accomplished when a group of community nurses are attached to a group of general practitioners, both being responsible for the same defined community of patients. The nurses and doctors records should be easily accessible to each other and regular meetings and discussions concerning the care of patients should be possible.

The second aspect to be considered is concerned with the treatment room nurse or the practice nurse. She does not normally have any responsibility for providing nursing care in the patient's home. She is, however, accessible to patients who are seeking nursing rather than doctor care in the practice, and in most instances, she has a special responsibility for health education and prevention.

The role of practice nurses is only now beginning to be clearly defined and their potential in case finding and health education and surveillance has not yet been fully explored. They can contribute to prevention with immunization programmes. In some practices the nurse has a computer terminal in her office so that she has ready access to information concerning the immunization state of the patients consulting her and has access to their health profiles. She can therefore actively contribute to case finding and identify vulnerable patients in the practice. In some situations, however, her role has become much more active and she is available to undertake selective screening procedures.

She can play an important part in health education and in the provision of continuing care for patients with chronic disease. For example she can instruct asthmatics in the use of inhalers and teach them how to monitor their peak flow rates; she can teach diabetics how to monitor their blood glucose levels and advise patients with cardiovascular disease about low cholesterol or high fibre diets; and she can perform a wide variety of other tertiary preventive tasks.

Health visitors

There is a group of nurses who have had special training in prevention and health promotion and they are called health visitors. Ideally they are attached to doctors' group practices so that their responsibilities are coincident in terms of population with those of the doctors and the practice and community nurses. This provides what is described as the primary care team. It comprises a variety of professionals with a variety of well defined roles. In the ideal situation these roles are determined by the needs of the population for whom care is being provided. Inevitably resources do not always balance needs and members of the team must be prepared to exchange roles in response to demand. Restrictive practices, in the context of the primary care team, are detrimental to good care.

Health visitors have a special part to play in prevention and health education. In the provision of antenatal care they should meet all expectant mothers and advise them not only in terms of the medical aspects of their pregnancy, such as diet and exercise but also in terms of their statutory rights, such as maternity benefits. They have a statutory duty to visit all newborn infants within 14 days of delivery, and to monitor the development of these infants by carrying out regular developmental checks at 6 weeks, 7 months, 2 years, and 3½ years. They organize the routine immunization of infants and keep careful records using either card indexes or practice computers. They are concerned with health education in all age groups and should be accessible to doctors and patients seeking advice on such diverse problems as family planning, marital breakdown, the menopause, and retirement. In the provision of health care there is a need for individuals who have a primary commitment to health education and health promotion. In the context of the primary care team health visitors work closely with practice nurses.

Patient participation

Good general practice depends on a contract between the patient and the primary care team that identifies the responsibilities and the expectations of both partners to this contract. One attempt to develop the progress of this partnership and increase efficiency has been the development of patient participation groups.

The primary care team has a limited amount of time in which it can be freely accessible to the patient in the practice. Within any given practice there are immense human resources and there is immense human need. Can the general practitioner in some way resolve these problems by developing patient participation groups? In such groups, patients can provide constructive criticism of the way in which services are provided and can explore ways in which the community of patients in the practice could contribute to the overall care of the population. With an ageing population and a worldwide reduction in hospital services, some solutions are needed that will embrace the very considerable resources in any community if they are to be harnessed to provide for the sick and disabled.

To limit the dialogue to the patient and the primary care team would ignore the role of the many other health professions who are involved with the promotion of health in primary care. Links must be made with hospital services, community social services, and local authority health clinics. When developing coherent programmes of health promotion it is necessary to involve all those concerned with the provision of primary health care. Ensuring good communications is one of the major problems in developing complex and sophisticated primary health care and health promotion.

CONCLUSION

There are enormous opportunities for doctors working in general practice to contribute to health promotion and prevention. General practice has, however, developed as a demand led activity in which doctors have responded to the problems presented to them by patients. Undergraduate and graduate training has been deficient in prevention and health promotion. There is a need for a change in the attitudes of both educators and future general practitioners. A change in attitude, however, will not produce major changes in the process of delivering care and outcome of care unless this is supported by good information and good management. At the same time doctors must take their patients with them in changing the ways in which they deliver care and there is an important need for greater patient participation in the provision of primary care.

REFERENCES

D'Souza, M. F., Swan, A. V., and Shannon, D. J. (1976). A long term controlled trial of screening for hypertension in general practice. *Lancet*, i, 1228.

Morrell, D. C. (1971). Expression of morbidity in general practice. *British Medical Journal*, 2, 454–8.

Sackett, D. and Holland, W. (1975). Controversy in the detection of disease. *Lancet*, ii, 257–9.

Stott, N. and Davis, R. (1979). The exceptional potential for each primary care consultation. *Journal of the Royal College of General Practitioners*, 29, 201–5.

The South East London Screening Study Group. (1977). A controlled trial of multiphasic screening in middle age. *International Journal of Epidemiology*, 6 (4), 357–63.

Treatment

This book is not intended to be a textbook of general practice. The general principles concerning the treatment of patients in general practice will therefore be considered rather than the treatment of specific diseases. Many of these principles are equally applicable to the specialist, but the work of the general practitioner is so varied, both in content and context, and is much less specific in treatment, that it demands a particular appreciation of the personal relationships and environmental factors that contribute to treatment.

The most important therapeutic influences in general practice are the doctors themselves. They are prescribed in various doses at every consultation (Balint 1971). Much of this therapy is administered unconsciously. Only by careful analysis of the doctor–patient relationship can doctors determine the influence of themselves on their patients.

The 'Balint' seminars, established originally at the Tavistock Clinic in London, were designed to explore this area of human relationships. This technique has now been incorporated into training programmes for general practice throughout the world. Doctors are trained to look analytically at their patients' behaviour and their own response to this behaviour. They thus learn to recognize the dependent patient, the insecure and aggressive patient, and the uncooperative patient, and equally they learn to recognize when they themselves are illustrating these characteristics. In this way it is possible to obtain some insight into the psychodynamics of the consultation.

Listening

A proper understanding of the problems experienced by patients, and their response to these problems, enables doctors to provide for their patient's needs, which may simply be for advice or for a sympathetic ear. Of these two forms of treatment, listening is by far the most difficult, but it is sometimes prevented by lack of time. This often causes subsequent regret when doctors realize that they would have saved time in the long run if only they had listened to what their patients were trying to tell them. More often doctors fail to listen because they are too keen to ask questions and give advice.

Some patients need to be encouraged to talk. The doctor might achieve this by simply adopting a relaxed, open, posture and remaining silent, or by asking an open ended question, or by using some remark such as 'Tell me about it'. Sometimes the doctor might suspect that the patient needs to talk about a particular problem but finds it embarrassing or difficult to start. It may then be necessary to ask specific open questions about work, family, or sex. If patients become hesitant or suddenly stop they might be helped to continue by the doctor simply repeating the patient's last few words. For example:

Patient: 'By the time we get to bed I feel so tired all I want is to turn over and go to sleep.'
Doctor: ' "Turn over and go to sleep"?'

If a consultation becomes extended by therapeutic listening both the patient and the doctor might become anxious about the other patients in the waiting room. It is then tempting for the doctor to try to terminate the interview by offering advice or a prescription. It is better to share this anxiety with the patient, try to identify the problem they are jointly uncovering, and to leave the consultation open and resume it on another occasion, perhaps at a special appointment.

A little reflection will show any doctor the importance of being a good listener. It is something we are always looking for in others. When we have a problem we go to someone we respect to discuss it. We usually refer to this as going for advice. What almost invariably happens is that we subject our adviser to a monologue, make up our own mind what we should do, and then leave giving thanks for the advice given. If our adviser did all the talking we would be disappointed, and would almost certainly go elsewhere for advice in the future. This is often the situation of the patient who approaches the doctor for advice, but who, if given the chance, is invariably content to talk out the problem, and then leaves feeling much better. This is a very important function of general practitioners, but one about which they learn little as students. They are brought up to regard every patient contact as one requiring a diagnosis of organic pathology and a positive treatment. In looking for the diagnosis they might miss the very obvious one— that the patient wants to talk. They might then find themselves prescribing treatment that is inappropriate and excessive.

Advice

In some cases the doctor will, however, need to act positively. Reassurance, sympathy, support, advice, and encouragement might all be appropriate in different cases. The application of these in different circumstances may be illustrated from some of the cases already considered. Mrs L. (case 27), who had failed to consummate her marriage, was in need of specific advice. Mrs T. (case 34) needed reassurance, and Mrs D. (case 36) needed sympathy, which she failed to obtain from her doctor with serious results. Mrs V. (case 37) wanted somebody to talk to and so the doctor encouraged her to visit each week to tell him how things were getting on.

General practitioners will be asked for advice on a variety of subjects covering a wide field, which is by no means limited to medicine. Some of the requests will be outside their knowledge, but they must know where to direct their patients to obtain the requisite information. Much of the advice they will be asked to give will, however, be within their capability as educated men or women with experience of people, and will concern interpersonal relationships either in the home or at work.

In providing this advice it is important for doctors to try to visualize the patients' real problems. It is not sufficient for them to pontificate and tell them how they should live their lives. They must, in general terms, try to assess the significance of the various aspects of a problem, put these objectively to the patients, and allow them to make their own decisions. In all this they must try to avoid becoming emotionally involved with the patients. A specific case may illustrate these points.

Case 50. Mrs B., aged 28, complained to the doctor of tiredness. She had three children aged 5, 3, and 1 year. She said that her husband was unsympathetic and that he never took her out and often went out in the evenings drinking with his friends. He left her short of money, and at times became violent towards her. She felt that the doctor should give him a talking-to. The doctor, now roused to the sad predicament of Mrs B., began to regard Mr B. as an inhuman brute and arranged to interview him. Mr B. turned out to be quite human. He complained that his wife was an incompetent housekeeper. She became involved in debts, which he had to settle, and when he came home tired in the evening he found the home dirty, the children still running about, and no supper prepared for him. He agreed that he became violent towards his wife. Having heard both sides of the story, the doctor was less emotionally disturbed and less liable to offer unsuitable advice and was in a position to bring husband and wife together to discuss their problems and differences objectively.

Much of the advice that doctors provide is directed to modifying the patient's environment or way of life. In doing this they must realize the full implications of their advice. They should endeavour to set the objective facts, as far as they know them, before patients, and allow them to make up their own minds. 'Doctor's orders' should be avoided at all costs. Ill conceived doctor's orders have led to an immense amount of misery in life, as is well illustrated by case 11. If patients are unable to obey the orders they might well develop relationships with their doctors that are based on feelings of guilt or deceit, and to abide by some orders would take away all that is worth having in life! Changes of occupation are commonly recommended. In particular, patients are often told to get a lighter job, or to take life easy. Unfortunately, most of the really heavy jobs are carried out by men of limited intelligence who would find it impossible to hold down a job requiring more brain and less brawn. To tell a builder's labourer to obtain a lighter job would, in many cases, be completely unrealistic advice. In certain special cases patients may be registered as disabled, and in this way will receive assistance from the Department of Social Security in obtaining suitable employment. In the case of young people it is often possible to arrange a course of industrial rehabilitation when their aptitudes can be tested and suitable employment secured. In many cases, however, when patients have been advised to change their occupation, careful consideration discloses that the advice given was unnecessary. Many patients who have previously been regarded as permanent invalids after an acute illness are found, after proper treatment and ample time for convalescence, to be capable of returning to their former occupation. Illnesses such as myocardial infarction, pulmonary tuberculosis, and diabetes should preclude very few people from resuming their previous jobs.

This aspect of medical advice has been particularly stressed because it is one about which doctors often give insufficient thought, and consequently place their patients in positions in which they have to either ignore the advice given or put themselves into an untenable situation. General practitioners should have inside knowledge about the type of employment that their patients undertake. By visiting factories in their area they can gain insight into the full implications of certain jobs in terms of the physical effort required and the financial reward. This relationship with industry will greatly facilitate the rehabilitation of an employee after illness. Such a relationship is a good investment for all concerned. It is greatly appreciated by the worker who is genuinely ill, and it acts as a deterrent to the shirker who can be a source of great frustration to doctor and management.

Rest

Advice concerning occupation is only one aspect of the even more commonly issued directives prescribing rest. There has been a fall in recent years in prescriptions for bed rest, and the dangers of confining a patient to bed for any long period are being increasingly appreciated. This is particularly so in the elderly, when there are risks of thromboembolism, stiffening joints, muscle weakness, and osteoporosis. Even young people find it difficult to be left peacefully in bed for more than a few days, and the results of early ambulation, particularly following surgery, have fully justified this attitude.

It is questionable whether this has been carried too far in cases of acute illness. Patients with tonsillitis, gastro-enteritis, or bronchitis are commonly treated with antibiotics and encouraged to remain ambulant. It is extraordinary how little is known about the benefits that accrue from rest in bed, but bowel and throat infections might recover more quickly if the patients remain in bed. A little more bed rest and rather less antibiotic treatment might achieve quicker resolution of many of the acute infective ailments with which doctors are presented. For economic reasons, the breadwinner in a family will often prefer to remain ambulant when ill, and a mother will rarely be able to indulge in such luxury as bed rest.

Rest, other than in bed, is often requested by patients. The expression 'I feel I need a good rest' is very common. Rest, which implies wandering around aimlessly at home and sitting in front of the television, is necessary in the phase between bed rest and return to work, but is rarely of value to the patient who asks for a 'good rest'. Diagnosis in these cases must precede treatment. Usually a temporary change of occupation and, if possible, environment is required. The housewife might need to get away from her home and children, or the business man away from an over-demanding business. Surprisingly, this type of request rarely comes from the manual worker who might well need a rest, or from the truly overworked housewife. It is much more commonly requested by the office worker who spends far too much time sitting about and who often eats too much. In this case the right prescription might be violent exercise, preferably out of doors. The other group who often make this request are housewives who are under, rather than over, worked. They are usually suffering from boredom and what is needed is a prescription that takes them out of their self-centred, uninteresting lives, and gives them some demanding and worthwhile employment.

Exercise

Nowadays, when the possession of a car, a television, and a telephone makes it almost unnecessary for most people to have any built-in method of progression, advice on exercise is often more important than the encouragement of rest. In certain types of middle-class practice doctors should bear this in mind. Their patients might look askance when they recommend that they should walk to work or indulge in 15 minutes skipping each day to cure their tension headaches, but this prescription is cheap, has few side effects, apart from a little muscular stiffness, and above all works.

Exercises designed to strengthen certain muscles or move certain joints may also be desirable. In the early treatment of chronic bronchitis and asthma, teaching the patient breathing exercises and encouraging plenty of outdoor exercise will do more good than any drugs. The chronic backache suffered by many women as the result of the unhealthy posture demanded by so many household tasks, responds well to regular exercise or swimming.

Diet

Advice on diet is often requested, particularly by women, and is often even more desirable in both sexes. In the treatment of many conditions, such as osteoarthritis and hypertension, it is necessary for the patient to lose weight. It is now well established that patients who get fat might eat no more than their slender siblings; their metabolism is merely different. Thus individuals who have a tendency to become fat cannot simply diet for a period of time to reduce weight but must develop a life-long change in their eating patterns. To simply produce a diet sheet is usually valueless. Patients must be convinced that they have to adopt a different life-style; short-term dieting is a waste of time for doctors and patients because they will return to their pre-diet weight as soon as they stop the diet.

There are some environmental stresses that cause patients to eat excessively and it is important to identify them. Excessive eating might be due to boredom or be used as a sedative, and an appreciation of this will help in the management. A full history of the patient's eating habits should be taken, and this should be followed by a full explanation of the seriousness of obesity for this individual, and instruction of the principles of weight reduction. This must be tailored to suit each individual case. The patient may then decide whether he or she wants to reduce their weight. A diet sheet that is simple and interferes as little as possible with the patient's way of life may then be given. If anorectic drugs are used, it must be explained that their only action is to reduce the appetite and thus relieve some of the suffering involved in weight reduction.

Dietetic advice may be required in diseases other than those made worse by obesity, of which diabetes is the main example. Providing the patient with a diet that is simple and will not inconvenience the whole household is most important. Most patients, if they can understand why a particular diet is necesary and how they can adhere to it with minimal inconvenience, will be happy to co-operate. Very few will persist on a diet simply because it is 'doctor's orders'. Nearly all special diets involve added expenditure on food and this is something that should always be considered and explained to the patient. In some cases, such as old age pensioners, the Department of Social Security will give an extra allowance to patients needing dietetic treatment, and such people should be encouraged to take advantage of this.

Smoking and alcohol

These are two subjects that are targets for medical prohibition. Alcohol in moderation is probably a useful drug. It is used as a relaxant at the end of a stressful day and to facilitate social contact. It may be taken in excess by those who can afford it without producing serious social problems, but with important physical consequences. More importantly, alcohol is a cause of serious social disorder. Within the family it is often associated with violence, with poverty due to excessive expenditure on the drug, and with crime due to drinking and driving and intemperate behaviour. In general practice advice concerning alcohol intake is therefore most often given in the context of counselling in relation to the family or the individual work record or criminal behaviour. Information concerning the physical risks of excessive alcohol is part of the general practitioner's preventive role, and is important in the management of gastrointestinal disorders and liver disease. A total ban on alcohol is only rarely justified.

Smoking is now widely accepted by the public as being detrimental to health. Adult smokers usually feel guilty about their habit and their inability to break it. They often need and want help, but they might react angrily to pontifical statements. It is common for the apostolic zeal of young general practitioners as health educators to undermine potentially promising doctor–patient relationships when a gentler approach would be more productive. Attempts to reform pensioners, who have survived to this age despite their apparently unhealthy lifestyles, are usually doomed to failure. The important problem concerning smoking is how to prevent the development of this addiction in adolescence when peer pressure still seems to exert an irresistible influence.

Explanation

The delicate balance between what is medically desirable and what is good for the individual patient is very difficult to maintain. It is, however, the duty of general practitioners. It is they who, by their knowledge of their patients, are in a position to weigh up the pros and cons of each case. The cardiologist might, for example, say that this patient should never have a baby. Medically this might be correct, but the family doctor might know that having a child means more to this individual than anything in the world. It is his or her duty to put all the facts to the couple concerned, but to leave the decision to them, and if this is contrary to the specialist's advice, to support them in their high endeavour. After all, if the only consideration is the preservation of life, doctors should prohibit all their patients from rock climbing. Many people, however, knowing the risks involved, are happy to indulge in this hazardous exercise for the physical and emotional rewards they derive from it. Some patients will be called on in the course of their lives to undertake tasks or responsibilities that endanger their health. If they still decide that it is right for them to proceed the doctor may regard them as foolhardy, but should always be in a position to admire their courage and give them every support.

Under the heading of advice comes the general practitioner's role of explanation. There are many diseases for which no treatment is necessary, and others where none is available. Here there is nothing to offer but explanation. Even in diseases responsive to treatment, a few words of explanation are of great therapeutic value. Letters from hospital specialists often conclude by saying that the patient was reassured. It is often a comfort to know that there is no organic disease to account for a particular symptom and it may be sufficient to produce a cure. If, however, the symptom persists, the patient is driven to conclude that either the specialist has made a mistake, or the symptom is a figment of the imagination. It is then important for the family doctor to discuss the whole problem with the patient, and explain that such symptoms might be caused by disorders of function that cannot be objectively demonstrated. This might be a suitable time to start a full psychotherapeutic approach, but the doctor should always give the patient an opportunity to voice fears, and to discuss the significance of his or her complaint.

Explanation is equally important in diseases that require further investigation or treatment. It must be worded to suit the individual's intelligence. This task, which is so often neglected, falls to family doctors. They should never assume that it has been done by somebody else. Whatever the outcome of treatment, their patients will always be grateful that they have shown an interest in their problems and have appreciated the implication of their disability. Patients vary in their ability to comprehend medical jargon, and much of what is said to them is often quite beyond their understanding. This is often the cause of the 'uncooperative patient'. Nobody can be expected to persist in time consuming tests and discomfort unless he or she understands why it is necessary. If patients can be fully convinced of the value of a certain line of treatment, they will rarely fail to co-operate.

Minor illness and self-medication

General practitioners have an important educational part to play in helping patients deal with minor illness without seeking medical care. I have shown that over 50 per cent of symptoms experienced by patients lead to some form of self-medication, while only 3 per cent lead to consultation with a doctor (Morrell and Wale 1976). During consultations doctors might reassure patients who have tried to manage their illnesses before consulting by telling them that they have behaved appropriately. By contrast, doctors might tell those who have not tried home remedies but have rushed to them for advice that perhaps they could have managed on their own. An experiment in which my group practice provided a random sample of patients with a booklet describing the significance of some common symptoms of illness, how these could be managed in the home, and when it is appropriate to seek medical advice, led to a fall in demand for care in these patients compared with a control group (Morrell *et al.* 1980).

Psychotherapy

It is clear that no doctor can practise medicine without carrying out some psychotherapy. What is being considered here, however, is not the therapy that occurs unconsciously at any doctor–patient contact, but a line of treatment based on a psycho-analytical diagnostic approach. One of the greatest difficulties facing general practitioners is determining the limit to their field of work. If they expand this field in one direction they must almost certainly restrict it in another. A doctor faced with a patient suffering from anaemia has three alternatives. Firstly, the doctor can, with the help of a laboratory, diagnose the precise cause of this condition and treat it appropriately. Alternatively, on detecting a low haemoglobin concentration the doctor might refer the patient at once to a physician, and finally, the doctor might go part of the way along the diagnostic road, elucidate that the patient is suffering from an iron deficiency anaemia, prescribe appropriate treatment, and only when this fails, summon the aid of a specialist. The doctor's knowledge of anaemia and the time available will be the main factors determining the course of action taken.

The same principles apply in the psychiatric field, but with two important reservations. Very few general practitioners have the requisite knowledge to undertake psychotherapy whereas most have been trained to deal with anaemia. The treatment of mental illness is, on the whole, more time consuming than treating physical disorders. For these reasons doctors might feel tempted to refer patients with mental illness to a specialist. Unfortunately, few psychiatrists will be prepared to undertake psychotherapy with patients. There are some who feel that this is an essential part of general practice. They encourage doctors to look past the soma at every consultation and recommend a detailed analysis of the personality beyond. They carry the diagnostic process much further than has been suggested in this book. Others, on the contrary, see a danger in this. 'Should we look for Psyche under every bed, and if she is there should we always drag her out, strip off her garments and parade her naked before the patients, who may or may not have known of her presence?' (Batten 1964).

It is clear that the relationship that develops between general practitioners and their patients offers unique opportunities for psychotherapy. There are, however, very few doctors with the necessary skills to indulge in this work. The psychotherapeutic relationship is not without risk, and to establish this without the knowledge required to see it through might only increase the patient's anxiety, or place either patient or doctor in an untenable position from which they can only withdraw by breaking their relationship altogether.

It is very important for general practitioners to look beyond organic disease and to be prepared to diagnose mental illness in a positive way. If they have the aptitude and the time they might learn to provide a form of psychotherapy that will help their patients to adapt to the strains that they are encountering in their lives without using an excessive amount to time. This has sometimes been described as the 'listening' treatment. This demands time but not a great deal of specialized skill. The ability to listen non-judgementally, to ask appropriate questions, to encourage the patient to seek an answer to their problems without suggesting solutions, should be within the skills of all general practitioners. Increasingly, clinical psychologists are providing services in general practice, either by attachment to group practices or through referral to hospital clinics. They provide a variety of behavioural therapies, particularly in the field of phobic anxiety states, and they can increase the resources of the primary care team.

Use of drugs

In a book of this size, it is impossible to consider treatment of illness in any detail. This section is included to provide some general principles that govern the management of common symptoms encountered in general practice. Two areas of treatment will be considered in this section. Firstly, the use of antibiotics in the management of infection, and secondly, the treatment of some common symptoms of illness.

Antibiotics

Of the curative drugs, antibiotics are the most important and account for 25 per cent of general practitioners' drug bill. They have done more than anything in the last two decades to revolutionize general practice. General practitioners no longer have to impotently look at patients with pneumonia, otitis media, pelvic inflammatory disease, etc. They can now cure these diseases. In fact they have become so easy to cure that there is a tendency to forget they were ever a problem. The 'interesting case' of thirty years ago has become quite uninteresting.

The efficiency of general practitioners in curing infective diseases is one of the reasons why they are in such demand by their patients. They know the curative power at doctors' disposal and demand this in both suitable and inappropriate conditions. In addition, doctors preserve the lives of many patients who do not have the natural resistance to survive to adulthood unaided, and who are likely to need the continued support of a physician throughout life.

It is sometimes said that general practitioners use antibiotics unnecessarily. This is probably also true of hospital doctors, and the use of them must be constantly reviewed. There are many aspects to this problem. General practitioners often use antibiotics simply because they are family doctors, that is they are doctors working in the family and in the home. It calls for little courage to leave a child with bronchitis in a hospital bed under the watchful eye of a ward sister knowing that the doctor will be informed of any sign of deterioration in the patient's condition. To leave such a child under the anxious eye of his or her mother, often a very uncritical eye, is less easy. This can of course be abused, and sometimes antibiotics are left to relieve the general practitioner's anxiety in inappropriate situations.

Many of the conditions in which the general practitioner uses antibiotics do not readily lend themselves to bacteriological examination before treatment, for example, otitis media, or bronchitis and pneumonia in children. In others, however, they can control their treatment more rationally if they have the services of a bacteriologist. These services are now available to most general practitioners, although those working in country districts might have transport problems. Despite this, the number of doctors who regularly use these services is small. The time involved in taking a bacteriological specimen from a patient and then conducting it to the laboratory creates a problem, and the sheer size of this problem in times of an epidemic is very considerable. There is little doubt that if bacteriological examination was conducted on every patient with a sore throat or diarrhoea the present laboratory service would break down. Doctors must always ask themselves how bacteriological examination will influence their treatment.

In many circumstances, doctors will compromise between the ideal and the practical; they will initially treat many infections on the basis of probability, and call on the bacteriologist only in those cases that fail to respond to treatment. The question of whether to use antibiotics in many of the simple infections seen in general practice is still a vexing one. In tonsillitis, for example, most cases clear up without antibiotics and without serious complications. Recovery, however, is quicker if the patient is treated with penicillin. Doubtless those doctors who contend that the virtual eradication of rheumatic fever from the community was related to the introduction of penicillin will prefer to treat a large number of patients unnecessarily rather than miss one who really needs an antibiotic. It has also been elegantly shown that social factors play a part in determining whether doctors use antibiotics in the treatment of tonsillitis (Howie 1976).

In acute bronchitis, general practitioners tend to prescribe antibiotics if the cough is productive of purulent sputum. It has, however, been shown that in young people, in the absence of abnormal signs in the chest, recovery from such an illness is uninfluenced in the short term by the use of antibiotics (Stott and West 1976). Whether such treatment influences the ultimate development of chronic bronchitis is much more difficult to determine.

Chronic bronchitis is another disease where there is some difference of opinion on the correct use of antibiotics. Trials have shown the value of long-term tetracycline treatment in these patients, but this is not universally accepted and many doctors limit treatment to acute exacerbations.

The importance of providing patients with adequate doses of antibiotics and continuing them for an adequate period must be stressed. This often presents problems for general practitioners. If antibiotics have to be administered by injection, doctors will either have to see patients daily or call on the services of district nurses. A greater problem, however, is ensuring that patients continue to take the drugs once they feel better. This must be insisted on when the prescription is issued, and subsequently reinforced. If doctors calculate the length of treatment and provide a supply just sufficient to cover this, they can then insist that patients take all the tablets provided and check whether there are any left at the end of treatment. Giving a patient a prescription is, of course, no guarantee that the treatment will be taken, as the following case illustrates.

Case 51. Mrs Y., brought her 2 month old daughter to the doctor with a discharging ear. A swab from the ear grew a haemolytic streptococcus, and so the mother was given a bottle of penicillin V suspension. The mother assured the doctor that the child was taking it well from the spoon, but 5 days later another swab from the ear again grew the haemolytic streptococcus. Mother was further questioned about the administration of the medicine and she assured the doctor that baby was taking it well, but admitted that vomiting occurred after each dose. Subsequent treatment with penicillin by injection was entirely satisfactory.

Case 52. Mrs B's child, Jacqueline, aged 4 years, was suffering from bronchitis. The doctor prescribed ampicillin syrup. Three days later, when he visited, Jacqueline was up and about and Mrs B. pronounced her cured. The doctor commented that the medicine obviously suited Jacqueline and encouraged Mrs B. to continue treatment until it was finished. Mrs B. then admitted that she had not in fact got the prescription, but would do so on Friday when her husband gave her the house-keeping money.

When patients are irresponsible, and when treatment is a matter of great importance, it is often advisable to administer a drug by injection rather than depend on oral treatment. This also applies to patients who are likely to vomit.

Case 53. John G., aged 7 years, developed acute lobar pneumonia. The doctor was called at 9.00pm and provided the parents with a suspension of penicillin V. He had just arrived home at 11.00pm when Mrs G. telephoned to say that John had vomited his medicine. The doctor had no alternative but to revisit and give him penicillin by injection. He regretted that he had not foreseen this possibility 2 hours before.

Naturally, no doctor likes to inject children when this is avoidable, but there are many circumstances in which this is the best route for administering an antibiotic, having consideration for the patient's intelligence, reliability, and physical condition.

Symptomatic treatment

Most of the prescribing done by doctors is for drugs that will relieve certain symptoms without curing the underlying condition. This includes the relief of symptoms caused by minor self-limiting illness and the very large group of chronic incurable diseases that cause much ill health in society. This important aspect of medical care is sometimes neglected in doctors' training, which tends to focus on their curative role.

Symptoms presented to doctors usually concern some form of distress that is experienced by the patient. The commonest form of distress is that due to pain, and the lives of many people are made miserable by pain that could be relieved. Some do not consult the doctor, and this might be for a variety of reasons. They might accept pain as an inevitable accompaniment of the ageing process. They might fear that pain indicates life-threatening disease, the presence of which they prefer to deny. They might be afraid that consultation will lead to operative treatment, which they wish to avoid. Other people go to doctors, but, because they cannot cure the underlying cause, they feel frustrated and unable to help, and do not really apply themselves to the problem of pain relief.

The treatment of pain

As in other forms of treatment the most important factor in achieving success is diagnostic accuracy. The precise cause of the pain must be ascertained. This applies not only to those patients who are suffering from some acutely painful condition such as gout or a tennis elbow, when the correct treatment will almost invariably produce relief, but also to the so-called chronically sick, when there is a danger that the doctor will regard pain as an inevitable part of some degenerative or neoplastic process, amenable only to analgesics.

In approaching this problem it is helpful to consider the various methods that may be employed in different circumstances. Modifications of the patient's life might be all that is required to relieve pain that would otherwise be incapacitating. This is particularly true in pain produced by exercise, such as intermittent claudication or cardiac pain, when a change in job, or a change in location of the patient's home, might be all that is necessary. The housewife with osteoarthritis of the knee may be spared a lot of pain by reorganizing her day so that she spends less time standing. Some modifications of the kitchen furniture will often do more for her than a prescription for analgesics.

Attention to household furniture and the acquisition of specially designed handles, cutlery, and various tools are of particular value to patients with rheumatic or neurological disorders. This approach to the problem of rehabilitation is very much the affair of general practitioners. Some patients benefit from a period of treatment in a progressive physical medicine or orthopaedic department, but there are many more patients who continue to suffer because general practitioners are either not aware of the facilities available or do not consider whether this therapeutic approach would be advantageous.

There are many specific forms of pain that will respond to specific therapeutic measures. If such pain presents as a new symptom in a previously healthy individual it is likely to be investigated and treated on its merits. Such specific measures might be overlooked in patients in whom a diagnosis of incurable disease has already been made, and who have, as it were, been given up as hopeless. Family doctors must be on the guard for this situation. The natural history of most chronic disorders reveals periods of activity and progression, alternating with relatively quiescent periods. The specialist might have nothing to offer a patient with generalized osteoarthritis, but a flare-up in a single joint might call for a renewed therapeutic endeavour, varying from local heat treatment to steroid injections or even complete surgical arthrodesis. Likewise, the patient with inoperable carcinoma might be relieved of a lot of suffering by local radiotherapy when secondary deposits in the bone subsequently develop.

Doctors must constantly review treatment in these chronic disorders, and must not be afraid to call in a variety of specialists to deal with any new problems that arise. In doing so, they will often be able to give patients not only relief from pain but also the comfort of knowing that they have not just been put on one side as incurable, and it will postpone the day when all the doctor can offer is analgesics.

The intelligent use of analgesics is one of the hallmarks of good general practitioners. This is an area of medicine in which they have special experience and should become experts. With the advent of powerful curative drugs like antibiotics, it is easy to forget that many acute inflammatory conditions are very painful. In the enthusiasm to prescribe the specific remedy, it is easy to fail to prescribe a drug to relieve the pain that will continue to be experienced until the specific remedy takes effect. In treating acute otitis media, pleurisy, or a pulp infection of the finger, to cite a few examples, adequate analgesia during the first 48 hours will ensure a rested and satisfied patient, and will also be reflected in a fall in the number of emergency calls. Drugs of the aspirin group may be sufficient to relieve the pain of these conditions, but if they are not, there need be no fear of prescribing more powerful remedies, such as pethidine or methadone, in illnesses that are short-lasting, but nevertheless, often acutely painful.

Acute traumatic conditions are also treated inadequately in terms of pain relief. X-ray of the damaged part and reassurance that there is no bone injury will not ensure that the patient has a night's sleep. Many of these conditions resolve quickly, but a powerful analgesic for one or two nights will increase the patient's comfort. Some more persistently painful contusions, such as bruised ribs or haematoma of the thigh muscle, might need regular analgesia over a long period. As many of these patients are initially treated in hospital, with their subsequent supervision being left to the general practitioner, there is a risk that they may fall between the two and their needs, in terms of pain relief, are often neglected.

By contrast, a very large quantity of analgesics is prescribed for patients suffering from ill-defined and often essentially functional disorders. Pain is a respectable symptom to present to the doctor, and it may take an infinite variety of forms, of which headache and backache are the most common. These are difficult symptoms to assess, and can indicate anything from a cerebral tumour to an unhappy love affair. The provision of analgesics will do nothing to mitigate the effects of the latter, and it is incumbent on the general practitioner to make as complete a diagnosis as possible. To eliminate the possibility of organic disease as a cause of pain, but continue to prescribe analgesics over a long period, is illogical. A more positive approach to the emotional factors or personality problems that are driving the patient to the doctor will, in the long run, prove to be an economical use of time, drugs, and energy expended in such a frustrating relationship.

In anticipating this situation it is advisable for doctors to encourage patients to see that symptoms may be caused by disorders of a functional nature as well as by structural damage, at an early stage in a consultation. If an exhaustive search is made for organic disease and patients are introduced to the concept of a functional disorder only when this has been excluded, they might have difficulty in accepting this as a cause of their symptoms and co-operating in further enquiry. If, however, taking the symptom of headache as an example, patients are allowed to consider the possibility that their symptoms might be due to emotional tension, at the same time and in the same way as they consider hypertension, sinusitis, or migraine as aetiological factors, any subsequent discussion of emotional factors will be facilitated.

In a large number of chronic diseases the doctor will ultimately be called on to give analgesics. This is particularly so in the chronic rheumatic disorders and in the later stages of malignant disease. In conditions such as osteoarthritis it is helpful to explain clearly to the patient the rational use of drugs in relieving pain. Diseases of this type are subject to exacerbations and remissions. They are often troublesome at particular times of the day, and the use of an anti-inflammatory analgesic half an hour before rising might be more valuable in terms of pain relief than much larger doses taken later in the day. It is very depressing to suffer from an incurable and painful complaint, and attention given to the individual's problems will be much appreciated and will often make it easier to bear pain that is inevitable.

There is a wide choice of analgesics for use in mild or moderate pain, but none of them is completely free from side effects. Aspirin has stood the test of time. It is both anti-inflammatory and analgesic. Some gastrointestinal blood loss occurs in most patients who take it regularly. Soluble forms of aspirin are just as likely to produce blood loss, but enteric coated aspirin and an acid stable compound of aluminium oxide and aspirin (Palaprin Forte) do seem marginally better in this respect. Paracetamol is a somewhat less powerful analgesic, but has fewer gastrointestinal side effects, although is more dangerous in over-dosage. Codeine and dihydro-codeine are effective but tend to cause constipation. Dextropro-poxyphene is effective but dosage over a long period may cause dependence. Whichever preparation is chosen, it is important to prescribe an adequate dosage. In addition to taking special care to avoid prescribing analgesics likely to exacerbate intercurrent dis-orders, for example, peptic ulceration, it is important to bear in mind drug interactions, such as that between aspirin and anti-coagulants or oral hypoglycaemic agents.

A large number of anti-inflammatory drugs that have an analgesic effect have been introduced. These include preparations such as indomethacin, which are particularly valuable in the man-agement of chronic arthritis but which have a tendency to cause gastrointestinal ulceration and bleeding, and may rarely be im-plicated in blood dyscrasias. They must therefore be used with discretion.

Treatment of cough

This is the most common symptom presented in general practice. The decision as to whether the patient is suffering from a significant lower respiratory infection, demanding antibiotic treatment, has already been discussed. Large numbers of cough remedies are available to the general public for symptomatic treatment, but many are expensive and few have been shown to be of real value. Linctus pholcodine or linctus codeine are prescribable and are of value in painful unproductive coughs. Most of the more complex formulations of cough remedies are not prescribable under the National Health Service, but pharmacists will advise patients on their purchase. Steam inhalations can be particularly helpful in dry, painful, coughs caused by laryngitis and tracheitis and the value of these inhalations may be increased by the addition of menthol or eucalyptus. In recurrent night cough in children, the possibility of asthma should always be considered and some children will respond dramatically to salbutamol syrup administered at night.

Treatment of rashes

In these cases a definitive diagnosis is clearly important with the prescription of the appropriate treatment. The use of steroid preparations has revolutionized the management of primary irritant and allergic eczema. These preparations will, however, exacerbate rashes due to infection of bacterial or fungal origin. Many cases of primary irritant or allergic eczema are encountered in general practice and symptomatic treatment with a steroid preparation is often invaluable and justifiable in the absence of a clearly identifiable aetiological agent. In providing symptomatic treatment it is important to instruct the patient to consult again if the lesion does not resolve.

Treatment of diarrhoea

This is another very common presenting symptom in general practice. A history of travel abroad might indicate the need for bacteriological examination of the faeces. In children, management should centre round dietetic advice concerned with the withdrawal of all solid food and milk products for 24 hours, but with adequate hydration with simple fluids. Kaolin and morphine mixture can be purchased at the pharmacy and may be helpful in the management of acute diarrhoea in adults. If they do not respond to this, codeine phosphate 30 mg taken every 4 hours will usually produce symptomatic relief.

Treatment of vomiting

Most cases presenting in general practice are due to acute gastrointestinal infections or dietetic indiscretions. Many are accompanied by diarrhoea. An examination of the abdomen must always be undertaken in patients presenting with acute vomiting or diarrhoea, although this will usually be unhelpful. Symptomatic treatment is concerned with the complete withdrawal of food and frequent intake of small quantities of simple fluids. Kaolin and morphine mixture may be comforting.

Treatment of insomnia

It is always important to identify the cause of insomnia before prescribing treatment. If it is caused by some acutely stressful incident, such as an accident or a recent bereavement, short term management with night sedatives may be appropriate. More often it is a symptom of more serious mental illness when immediate symptomatic treatment may be inappropriate and may start a pattern of behaviour in which the patient becomes dependant on night sedation.

Treatment of anxiety and depression

These very common symptoms in general practice can rarely be resolved by symptomatic treatment. Acute anxiety due to some clearly defined incident such as an accident, burglary, or rape may require immediate symptomatic treatment with a tranquillizer such as diazepam. Acute depression, as presented in a grief reaction, may also need symptomatic treatment such as prescription of a night sedative. In most cases, however, a more detailed diagnostic approach must precede treatment.

Conclusion

Some of the common symptoms presented in general practice have been considered in this chapter. Of these, pain is by far the most common. In many cases symptomatic treatment is entirely appropriate, but this should be based on a clear definition of the patient's problem with, in many cases, a clear diagnosis of the underlying pathology and, in all cases, easy access to care if the problem is not resolved.

Continuing care in chronic diseases

About one half of all consultations in general practice are concerned with the provision of care for patients suffering from chronic disease. Some of these might develop relatively early in life, such as eczema, asthma, schizophrenia, diabetes, multiple sclerosis, peptic ulcer, or rheumatoid arthritis. Many, however, are associated with degenerative processes such as cardiovascular or cerebrovascular disease, osteoarthritis, chronic progressive neurological disorders, cancer, and senile dementia.

Role of the specialist and the general practitioner

In managing these conditions, it is important for undergraduates to understand the relative roles of the general practitioner and the hospital specialist. Exposed for the first time to general practice, they might be surprised to realize that the care of these patients occurs mainly in general practice. When viewed from the hospital setting, these disorders account for most of the out-patient and in-patient episodes of care, but these hospital episodes represent only a small part of the continuing care of these patients.

What then is the specialist's role in the care of these diseases? Very often the specialist will be involved in the initial diagnosis. Endoscopy might be required to confirm the diagnosis of a peptic ulcer, or colonoscopy to confirm the diagnosis of a carcinoma of the large bowel. In the diagnosis of important disabling diseases such as multiple sclerosis, rheumatoid arthritis, or senile dementia, there is a need for a second opinion, not just because the specialist can confirm the diagnosis and contribute to management but, more importantly, because the general practitioner can be provided with the support needed in treating a progressive disabling disorder. In some conditions, such as diabetes or asthma, an initial specialist assessment of the patient is often desirable so that a planned programme of care may be developed between specialist and general practitioner.

In the management of this group of diseases specialist skills will be required in a variety of ways and at a variety of stages in the natural history of the disease. In the diagnosis and surgical or palliative management of cancer, the specialist has an important part to play at an early stage in the disease; in the early management of coronary thrombosis or stroke, hospital care is often required; in the acute schizophrenic breakdown, hospital admission might be necessary; in the acute asthmatic attack that is resistant to conventional treatment, hospital admission will be required. The specialist's role in the management of these chronic disorders may therefore be summarized as being concerned with the initial diagnosis, with support for the general practitioner, with surgical intervention, and with the management of acute life-threatening episodes occurring in the course of the disease. Medical students will be familiar with all these situations, but will be unaware of the characteristics of the care provided between these episodes.

In the past there has been a tendency for the continuing care of patients with chronic diseases to be provided in hospital outpatient departments with the creation of large 'follow-up' clinics for patients suffering from diseases such as epilepsy, chronic bronchitis, or hypertension. Most of these disorders are best managed by a doctor who can review their care regularly, and as often as is necessary, in the community and who can relate this to their family and social resources. Today, general practitioners are expected to provide this care.

Setting strategies for care

Watkins (1980) pointed out that a major breakdown in determining standards of care in chronic diseases is the desire to produce quantifiable outcome measures that can be generalized to a group of patients who resemble each other only to the extent that they are labelled with the same common diagnosis. He showed that most patients suffering from one chronic disorder, such as diabetes or cardiac failure, also suffer from other disabilities that limit both their ability to comply with the care provided and to respond to treatment in a predictable way.

It is now fashionable to suggest that the outcome of care for such patients should be measured in terms of biochemical or functional parameters. Watkins' major contribution in this field was to point out that setting normal values in terms of outcome is pointless and that what is needed is an assessment for the individual patient in terms of what outcome can be realistically achieved. This means that in developing a strategy for the care of individuals suffering from chronic incurable diseases this strategy must be concerned with setting realistic objectives for the individual patient. They must take into account not just the whole range of disabilities the individual is experiencing but also the psychological and social factors that impact on the disease.

In developing a strategy for the management of chronic disease in general practice, it is helpful to separate the process of care from the expected outcome. It is often easy to identify certain process measurements in terms of the observations that should be made at predetermined intervals if optimal care is to be provided. An example of this was given in Chapter 4 in which a standardized medical record for the care provided for patients suffering from diabetes was described. The process of the care delivered can be measured against such a standard. It is, however, important to recognize that this might not equate with the outcome of the care.

Developing strategies for the care of individuals suffering from a variety of chronic diseases is an integral part of general practice. It must take into account the resources that are available to provide care. How often, for example, should the well controlled middle-aged hypertensive patient receiving treatment with beta-blockers be reviewed? Who should carry out this review, the doctor or the nurse? Increasing numbers of patients are being supervised in general practice for conditions such as raised blood pressure. It is important to use the resources available in the most cost-effective way to avoid care being given for some well recognized diseases at the expense of those suffering from conditions in which less organized therapeutic regimes have been worked out, but in which the patients none the less have important needs.

Multiple pathology and polypharmacy

With increasing age, individuals often develop a wide variety of diseases. Osteoarthritis commonly develops in association with ischaemic heart disease and cardiac failure. There might be concurrent hypertension, peripheral vascular problems, and peptic ulcer disease. Such patients might be receiving a wide variety of drugs that can interact with each other and with the multiple disease processes. In this example non-steroidal anti-inflammatory drugs may exacerbate peptic ulcer disease; beta blockers may impair peripheral vascular perfusion and exacerbate cardiac failure. Treatment in such cases must be tailored to the overall needs of the patient, bearing in mind not just side effects, but also drug interactions.

In the elderly, renal and hepatic function is often reduced and the excretion of drugs may be impaired. A dose of digoxin that may be satisfactory in a young person may cause toxicity in the elderly and may be fatal if combined with a potassium losing diuretic. In the elderly, new symptoms are commonly presented to the general practitioner that reflect, not the development of a new disease but the toxic affects of the treatment that the patient is receiving. New symptoms in patients receiving polypharmacy should always lead to a complete review of the drugs being prescribed, and in some cases it is desirable to gradually withdraw all treatment. In the presence of multiple pathology, there is a temptation to add a new drug to combat every new symptom presented without a proper review of the whole therapeutic regime.

Another reason for regularly reviewing treatment schedules is that disease is a dynamic process. A diagnosis might change with time and there is the risk that a patient labelled with a particular diagnosis will not be critically reviewed at regular intervals. Such a review is very necessary and it is desirable that patients receiving repeat prescriptions for chronic disease should be completely reviewed at least annually.

Psychosocial factors

In the management of chronic disease, psychosocial factors are of great importance. Many elderly and disabled live alone, often in housing estates where burglaries and muggings are day-to-day occurrences. They are frightened in their homes at night and sometimes frightened to leave their home during the day. This produces depression and agoraphobia, which influences the way in which they respond to their illnesses.

Clearly many patients would function more effectively if they had housing more suited to their needs, lived in more protected environments, or could be rehoused in warden-supervised housing complexes. Though general practitioners can draw the attention of social services and housing departments to the needs of individual patients, this is often unproductive as these services do not have the resources to respond. The doctor is therefore constrained to work within a socio-economic climate determined not by medical need but by political dictat. This is often very frustrating but none the less they must know about the social services available and how best their patients can avail themselves of these services.

In many parts of the country, social workers provide invaluable support for the chronically ill and disabled, evaluating their needs and providing services. These services include home helps. They visit the disabled daily to provide domestic services and do their shopping, but above all they provide a contact for the isolated patient, and daily supervision of their needs. Social services also provide a meals-on-wheels service in many areas, delivering hot meals to patients at mid-day. Here again, the regular contact with those who provide the service is as important as the service provided. In some cases alterations to housing can be made by the provision of modified toilet and bathing facilities, hand rails in the home, ramps for wheelchairs, etc.

These services are vitally important to those suffering from chronic incurable diseases and it is therefore important that the doctor responsible for their continuing care is the doctor working in the community, who is familiar with their homes and with the community services available.

Nursing care

The provision of adequate nursing care in the home forms an essential part of the continuing care of patients suffering from chronic disease. In many cases these nurses are attached to a particular general practice so that the doctors and nurses in the practice are responsible for the care of the same group of patients. This has enormous advantages in terms of day-to-day communications concerning the care of these patients. Community nurses are trained to visit patients in their homes and to assess their medical and social needs. These can then be discussed in the practice and a programme of care planned for individual patients, calling in the social services when necessary. Nurses supervise the medication of housebound patients, provide general nursing care in terms of hygiene, care of the bowels and bladder, dietetic advice, and specific nursing services. Such services include the administration of insulin to blind diabetics, treatment of varicose ulcers, and most importantly all the nursing requirements in the provision of terminal care.

In the case of single-handed general practitioners, it might not be feasible to attach a particular nurse to a practice and so the district nursing services are then based on a geographical area. In these situations the nurse will provide care for the patients of several doctors. The quality of communication and the planning of care that is then possible is inevitably much more difficult to ensure.

The management of chronic disease in general practice must be a team effort. On a day-to-day basis it involves the general practitioners, the district nurses, and the social services. On an episodic basis it involves specialists in the management of acute emergencies, demanding their special knowledge, skills, and hospital resources. Of paramount importance in all this is proper and effective communication between those providing care.

TERMINAL CARE

Terminal illness is often thought of as illness due to incurable cancer. In the population of patients for whom a general practitioner provides care, however, there are many patients who are terminally ill as a result of cardiovascular disease, chronic respiratory disease, progressive neurological disorders, and senile dementia. The provision of terminal care is not therefore restricted to the care of patients suffering from cancer, although they may present some of the most difficult problems. Communications between doctors and patients suffering from terminal illness have been discussed in Chapter 7. This chapter is concerned with the management of the symptoms and disabilities that occur in this situation.

Pain relief

Pain is an important problem in the management of many, but not all, terminal illnesses. Its appropriate management demands an accurate diagnosis of the cause of the pain, which will influence the sort of drugs that will be needed to control the symptoms. Consideration must also be given to the extent to which pain relief will cause drowsiness and the patient's own wishes in this respect.

Pain in malignant disease may be caused by direct involvement of pain sensitive structures such as the pleura and peritoneum. Relief of pain in these cases will demand the use of analgesics such as morphine. It may be caused by bony metastases in which case non-steroidal anti-inflammatory drugs and local radiotherapy may be valuable. It may be caused by pressure on nerve roots when local injections will be helpful. It may be caused by secondary metastases in the brain when high doses of steroids will be of value. Pain may be exacerbated by depression and antidepressants may sometimes help, or by anxiety and insomnia, which may be relieved by anxiolytics such as diazepam or chlorpromazine. The prescription for pain relief must therefore be related as precisely as possible to the needs of the individual patient.

There will be a stage in terminal illness when pain can no longer be relieved by the regular use of simple analgesics such as aspirin, paracetamol, or dihydrocodeine. Inevitably, in most cases, a decision to introduce more powerful analgesics must be made. A variety of drugs are available such as methadone, pethidine, pentazocine, and dipipanone. Unless there are special indications for these drugs, it is probably sensible to prescribe in the first instance morphine sulphate continus (MST), which can be taken twice daily by mouth. The dosage should be adjusted to ensure that the patient does not experience breakthrough pain. Doses usually start at 10mg twice daily, and can be increased until complete pain relief is experienced. Some doctors are frightened by the amount of the drug necessary to relieve pain, but doses in the region of 150mg twice daily are not uncommon and, even on this dosage, patients can function effectively. If pain does break through despite using the long acting morphine preparations, it may be treated by a shorter acting preparation such as elixir of morphine hydrochloride. Patients often get added security by having such a preparation available. If these preparations are not successful in controlling pain, morphine or diamorphine may be administered continuously by use of a 'pump'.

When bone pain is a problem, the addition of a non-steroidal anti-inflammatory drug such as naproxen twice daily may be helpful. Local radiotherapy may also be of special value in these cases and maintaining good communications with specialists in this field is essential in achieving good pain control in malignant disease. Some hospitals have special pain control clinics in which anaesthetists and radiotherapists work closely together and they provide an invaluable resource.

In using high doses of morphine, constipation is almost inevitable. Regular use of lactulose solution helps to keep the stools soft and this may be supplemented by a stimulant laxative such as bisacodyl. It is important not to allow severe constipation to develop and if necessary suppositories or enemas may be used. Nausea or vomiting may also present problems when taking morphine, and this can often be relieved by concurrent treatment with chlorpromazine, prochlorperazine, or metoclopramide.

Pain is not the only source of distress in terminal illness. Predictably, anxiety and depression are often present and may exacerbate the pain. The members of the primary care team have an important part to play in allowing patients to express their fears. These may centre on the dying process, fear of uncontrollable pain, or anxiety about relatives being left behind, or unresolved personal conflicts. Listening can be of immense therapeutic value. Morphine is a useful anxiolytic, but the addition of, for example, diazepam taken three times daily may be helpful. A night sedative may also help. If depression is a problem a sedative tricyclic antidepressant taken at night may be valuable. Dexamethasone is often used for its anti-inflammatory action in treating terminal cancer and is also useful in increasing a feeling of well-being and improving appetite.

Dyspnoea commonly presents problems in patients dying of chronic respiratory and cardiovascular disease. Domiciliary oxygen is important and in patients dying slowly of chronic obstructive airways disease an oxygen concentrator may be ordered, usually after consultation with a respiratory physician. These patients also sometimes benefit from having a nebulizer available at home.

The most important aspect of looking after patients with terminal illness is good nursing care, with good communications between all those providing care. Regular attention to bowels, bladder, mouth, and skin is incorporated in the term 'general nursing care' and most district nurses can call on laundry services for the incontinent, the loan of commodes, urinals, feeding cups, etc., to support the family's resources. The regular visits of a nurse also supports the morale of the carers in the family and as she goes about her nursing tasks, patient and carers will often unburden anxieties that remain unspoken to the doctor.

It is often difficult for undergraduates to learn about terminal care in the hospital setting. When learning in general practice, home visiting in the company of the district nurse presents a unique opportunity to learn about such care.

Prescribing in general practice

In response to patients' needs, general practitioners prescribe a variety of drugs. The prescriptions they write are then presented to a pharmacist. There appears to be very little training for general practitioners in the art of prescribing or in the skill of writing a prescription. Pharmacists complain bitterly of the illegibility of prescriptions and the ineptitude of doctors in prescribing the correct amount of drugs or frequency of administration.

When doctors prescribe it is incumbent on them to communicate to the patients the frequency of administration, the duration of treatment, and the possible side effects. It is negligent for them to write the prescription in handwriting that can possibly be misinterpretated by the pharmacist, and if doctors' handwriting is so bad they should print their prescriptions. It is, for example, easy for a pharmacist to misinterpret a badly written prescription for chlorpromazine as chlorpropamide, and the results of such an error could be life threatening. In rural areas a close relationship usually exists between pharmacist and general practitioner and any queries can be easily resolved. In city centres, however, patients may present their prescriptions to a wide variety of pharmacies and such a relationship might not exist.

The quantity of drugs prescribed is another important consideration in general practice. The problem of compliance has already been mentioned. Patients are more likely to be compliant if doctors supply just sufficient drugs for the period of treatment and are able to tell their patients to take all the drugs prescribed.

With the increasing number of drugs on the market, major problems are developing with drug interactions. Hypotensive drugs, for example, may cause depression, but tricyclic antidepressants may interact with hypotensives. The simple aspirin interferes with anticoagulant treatment, and diuretics with hypoglycaemic agents. Pharmacists spend 4 years in attaining a degree course before they can enter general pharmaceutical practice. They are kept up to date through their literature and to provide adequate and safe drug treatment it is important to establish a partnership between the general medical practitioner and the general pharmaceutical practitioner. Finally, it is perhaps appropriate to ask how general practitioners can remain up to date with their prescribing. They are visited regularly by representatives of drug companies who encourage them to use their latest products. General practitioners must learn to look critically at the claims of any new form of treatment. They must be able to interpret the results of randomized controlled trials of treatment so that they are not seduced into prescribing a new drug on the basis of inadequate evidence. They must be aware of the cost of the drugs they prescribe. They must be aware that the undesirable side effects of new drugs usually take 5–10 years to display themselves, for example thalidomide. They would indeed be well advised to be highly conservative in their prescribing habits and to recognize that a really effective advance in treatment, such as penicillin, chlorothiazide, or sodium cromoglycate, does not need a drug representative to sell it. General practitioners should have a small repertoire of drugs with which they are very familiar, and should add to it only after making a critical evaluation of any new drug.

REFERENCES

Balint, M. (1971). *The doctor, his patient, and the illness*, (2nd edn). Pitman Medical, London.

Batten, L. W. (1964). Stress in life and medical practice. *Journal of the Royal College of General Practitioners*, **7**, 320.

Howie, J. G. R. (1976). Clinical judgement and antibiotic use in general practice. *British Medical Journal*, **2**, 1061–4.

Morrell, D. C. and Wale, C. J. (1976). Symptoms perceived and recorded by patients. *Journal of the Royal College of General Practitioners*, **26**, 398–403.

Morrell, D. C., Avery, A., and Watkins, C. J. (1980). Management of minor illness. *British Medical Journal*, **1**, 769–71.

Stott, N. C. H. and West, R. R. (1976). Randomized controlled trial of antibiotics in patients with cough and purulent sputum. *British Medical Journal*, **2**, 556–9.

Watkins, C. J. (1980). Experimental research into the quality of medical care delivered to patients suffering from chronic disease. Unpublished PhD thesis. University of London.

Index

abdominal pain 46–7, 84–5
accessibility 12–19
adolescents 109, 127
advice 122–7
  on alcohol 127
  on diet 126–7
  on exercise 125–6
  on rest 124–5
  on smoking 127
alcohol 110, 127
anaemia 88, 91, 130
analgesics 136, 137, 138, 147
antenatal care 111–12, 117
antibiotics 131–4
anxiety 15, 55, 60, 140, 147, 148
appointment systems 62
aspirin 136, 138, 150
assistantships, clinical 23
asthma 139

babies 72, 92, 112
backache 48, 86–7, 126
bacteriology 91, 132
balance, disturbance of 51
Balint seminars 120
barium studies 84
beta blockers 143, 144
blood pressure 110
bowel function, disturbances of 47
breathing
  disturbance of 52, 148–9
  exercises 125
British Medical Association
  Medical Practices Committee of 8
bronchitis 133

cancer 100, 142, 146, 148
capitation 6
cardiovascular disease 148
care
  continuity of 56
  primary 5–11, 20
    antenatal 111–12, 117
    financing of 6–7

  organization of 7–9
  postnatal 112
  principles of 5–6
  sources of 7
  terminal, *see* terminal care
care teams, primary 3, 117, 148
case finding, opportunities 110
cervical cytology 112–13
chest
  examination of 83
  pain in 49
children
  coughs in 139
  examination of 92–3
  history-taking in 71–3
  injection of 134
  primary prevention in 108
  prognosis in 96
codeine 138
communication skills 53–5
  with the dying 99–103
  observation 54–5, 70
  in prognosis 103–6
  teaching of 3, 53, 56
  verbal 55–63
    approach to consultations 60–1
    facilitation 56
community nurses 7, 8, 116, 145–6
  see also district nurses
constipation 148
consultations
  analysis of 75, 114
  factors influencing likelihood of
    16–17
  general practitioners' approach to
    60–1
  potential of 114
  referral rates 76
contract, doctor's, with patient 99
contusions 137
coughs 45, 83, 139

dentists 7, 8
depression 15, 88, 97
  prevalence of 23